# His Strength In Me

# His Strength In Me

Discovering Joy While Providing Care
for a Loved One May Seem Difficult

But You Are Not Alone

*By Lyndy Downs*

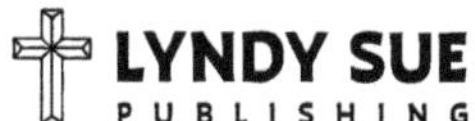

**His Strength In Me:**
Discovering Joy While Providing Care for a Loved One May Seem Difficult But You Are Not Alone
By Lyndy Downs



Cover by Nick Downs
Photography Credits: Tricia Lawley, Craig Fikse

Published by Lyndy Sue Publishing
lyndydowns.com



ISBN:
979-8-218-09321-1 (print)
979-8-218-09320-4 (ebook)

Printed in the United States of America
First Edition (2022)

In memory of my father, sister, brother, and all who bravely fought the battle against Huntington's Disease. So many lives were touched as a result of having known them.

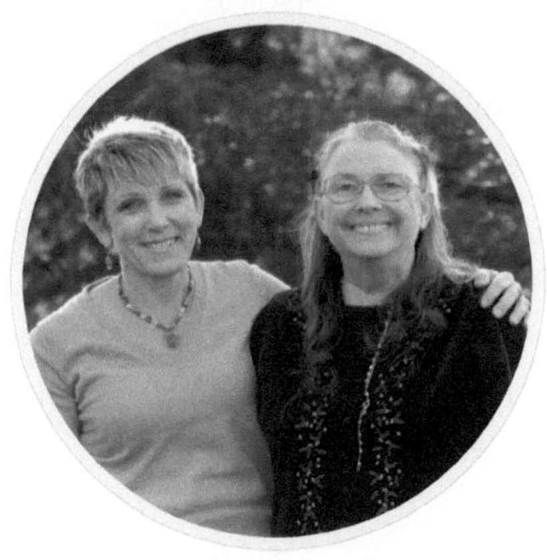

And in memory of my dear mom, one of the strongest people I have ever known. She gave me life in more ways than one. Her determination, love, and example provided an earthly foundation upon which to build. Without her, I would not be the person I am today. She lived striving selflessly to educate others and never gave up the fight for advancements in the study of Huntington's Disease and the hope of a cure.

# ACKNOWLEDGEMENTS

To my husband, Rob—thank you for championing my efforts in seeing this book to its completion. I am so thankful for you and our sons Cameron, Nick, and Michael, without whom I would not have been able to persevere during our family's battle with my mother's dementia. You showed God's love to Mom/Grandma and John despite the many required sacrifices.

An additional thank you to Nick—I just knew all those years of homeschooling would one day pay off! Seriously though, I thank God for gifting you with many talents and your willingness to use them on my behalf. I will never be able to thank you enough for the countless hours of research, support, and work as my publication agent, graphic designer, and marketing/distribution guru.

To all of my aunts, uncles, and extended family on both sides—thank you for always being there throughout my life, both emotionally and as my support network.

To Uncle Randy—I can never fully express how much your love, support, regular visits, wisdom, and advocacy on Mom's behalf meant to me. I know God used you mightily, in ways I could never fully express, in my life and hers.

In memory of my stepdad, John. I will always be grateful for his support and love for our family and my mom throughout the years.

To my friends who lifted me in prayer for so many years—
I am forever appreciative of the encouragement you gave me in some of my darkest moments.

To my dearest friend and adopted sister Julia—
thank you for your friendship, wisdom, insight, and ongoing support as I sought to make this book a reality.

To Martha, Vanessa, and Mary—
I gained much encouragement and insights along the way thanks to your input.

Special thanks to those who were part of the "nuts and bolts" in editing and publishing: Michelle, Toni, Kim, Lindsay, and Melissa. Your wisdom, expertise, and help were invaluable.

Finally, I thank my Lord and Savior, Jesus, for relentlessly pursuing me, loving me, and sacrificing Your life so that I would live. All glory and honor are Yours.

# TABLE OF CONTENTS

*...but those who hope in the LORD will renew their strength. They will soar on wings like eagles; they will run and not grow weary, they will walk and not be faint.*

*(Isaiah 40:31 New International Version)*

# Introduction

Since I was a child, I've believed in God's existence. However, as an adult, I realized that just believing in His existence wasn't enough. Instead of just knowing *about* Him, I needed to *know* Him. I needed to have a personal relationship with Him where I trusted He was and will always be who He says He is. I needed His grace, forgiveness, love, strength, and most of all, His gift of His one and only Son, Jesus Christ, as my Lord and personal Savior. My journey, and the road I followed, as a daughter, wife, mother, sister, and caregiver have all influenced my faith. However, I think it is in my weakest moments when I cry out to Him that God strengthens my faith in Him. It was and still is in those exact moments that I find myself genuinely searching for more of God.

For years I have thought about writing a book describing what it was like to grow up with Huntington's Disease in my family. Not only was I at risk for this disease, but I was also a caregiver, alongside my mother, for three members of my family who were afflicted with the disease. Yet, as all-encompassing as it was for much of my life, I eventually married, had three fantastic sons, and proceeded to live my "new" life outside of Huntington's Disease. The busyness of this life precluded me from acting upon my desire to write. However, after seventeen years of homeschooling, I "retired" with the thought of perhaps finally beginning the book. But a few months later, I would start another caregiving journey with my mother, who was diagnosed with Frontotemporal Dementia. After almost two years of caring for her in our home, we placed her in a memory care facility because we could no longer provide the required supervision and assistance she required. All these years later, God gave me enough nudges through sermons, several different book studies, and encouragement from friends and family to begin this book. Yet, I questioned how, when, and what I was to write.

Part of my inspiration came from an author I admire, Holley Gerth. Through her, I found assistance in a writing website entitled Compel and began my journey in writing this book. I gained my first boost by winning a writing challenge designed to craft an "elevator pitch." However, once I started learning some of the nuts and bolts involved in writing a book, I again questioned whether this was the path He wanted me to take. After all, I didn't know how to start a blog or gain a "following." He sent a dear friend into my life who encouraged me to create my page on Facebook, where I began my blog, entitled "More of Him, less of me." By now, one would think I would stop questioning His calling for me, but I didn't. He knew I needed more encouragement. A week or so later, as I sat chatting with a fellow volunteer about my desire to write, she told me that she was an editor. Her support and offer of assistance were the final boosts I needed. It still took several years and a few other supportive friends to make it through the book-writing and publishing process, but God is good and helped me see it through.

As I began the process, I was fortunate to have found copies of my old diaries, letters, papers, and several journals from my mother. These provided much of the insight I needed as I began to pen my story and subsequently became an integral part of this book. I know my mother would have wanted to share her story, as evidenced by the journal entry she wrote after a peer group session for people dealing with Huntington's Disease:

> *April 7, 1991* ———
>
> *I was asked whether talking about my past, and my losses was too painful or emotional. That's always a little difficult to answer. Of course, going thru it was painful...But, it seems the greater loss would be in not sharing some of those experiences with others that are going through similar happenings and perhaps feelings, with the hope that sharing [some of my experiences] might shine a little light into some of the corners shadowed by the unknown...[and], for me, make return visits to those 'corners' a little less dark, as well.*

Indeed, I hope that by sharing my experiences and those of my mother, you will find that you are not alone regarding the daily struggles, emotions, and feelings associated with caring for loved ones suffering from devastating diseases.

> *"Praise be to the God and Father of our Lord Jesus Christ, the Father of compassion and the God of all comfort, who comforts us in all our troubles, so that we*

*can comfort those in any trouble with the comfort we ourselves receive from God."*

*2 Corinthians 1:3-4*

It may have taken almost fifty years to accept that I needed God's strength to face these things, but that realization has been the most significant "aha" moment I have had in my entire life. My deepest desire is that my story will provide the same encouragement and hope I struggled to receive from God all that time and that you too will be able to see the hidden blessings amidst the turmoil. I pray that it will bring comfort and strength in times of hardship, whether as a caregiver for a loved one or in whatever trials this life may bring, so that you too may see His strength in you.

Lyndy

CHAPTER ONE

# The Calm Before the Storm

Some of my earliest and fondest memories are of my sister Chrysty, my brother Ronnie, and me going on road trips with our parents. We would take off across the U.S. in our Pace Arrow motorhome, complete with its vinyl-covered seats that I would always stick to, to visit relatives from both sides of the family. As we logged hundreds of miles across the long stretches of highway in the Southern and Midwestern states, my siblings and I reveled in the excitement of getting passing truckers to honk their horns from our perch glancing out the oversized back window. A favorite pastime was when our dad would stop at the chain of convenience stores called Stuckey's. He would let us choose a special treat and get his favorite peanut brittle. Sometimes, we traveled well into the night, eventually stopping at a rest stop. Then, after a good night's sleep, my dad would awaken early, as we still slept, and head out on the highway again. We would wake up to the sun shining in that big window, surprised that we were already back on the road to our next destination.

Once we arrived at Grandma Pearl's (my dad's mother) house in Kansas, we would have fun-filled afternoons with extended family. We dined on some of her specialties like sour watermelon-rind pickles and beirock, a German delight of dough filled with cabbage and ground beef, which became my favorite. My sister, brother, and I would spend days playing, and visiting with cousins, as we whiled away the time at the local Dairy Queen. I even remember heading to my aunt's house down the block and feeding sugar cubes to her horse.

Back home, I recall times of sitting in the backyard with my sister and playing with our Barbies. We had some of the most beautiful Barbie outfits because my aunt would make us handmade, one-of-a-kind designs, including wedding dresses made from material she had left from her gown. To this day, I have held on to some of those outfits, hoping that I can pass them along, with the fond memories they bring, to my granddaughters. Unfortunately, when you have all sons, Barbie clothes just aren't appreciated! We also enjoyed playing house and creating "casseroles" with the abundance of acorns from the neighbor's oak tree.

Holidays and birthdays were memorable as we regularly met at Poppo and Grammy's house (my mom's parents). I loved helping Grammy make her delicious homemade rolls. Unfortunately, no one can replicate them to this day, but one of my aunts has come close. Every Thanksgiving and Christmas, Grammy made her rolls, a large number and variety of pies, and a yummy cinnamon and sugar delight created from the leftover pie crust. During these gatherings, our family loved to play games. You could find Poppo rallying the attendees to join him in a few rounds of poker or horseshoes on any given occasion. We also enjoyed playing Yahtzee and Spoons. By all accounts, Spoons was the most active and competitive. I recall times when my mom and her sisters would wind up underneath the table trying to grab that last evasive spoon!

We would spend Easter Day hunting for dozens of colored, hard-boiled eggs. Of course, we had spent hours, in advance, dying and decorating said eggs. Inevitably, several of the creations, usually hidden by my dad, could never be found until days later when the dogs located them. We even had a live fluffy bunny waiting for us one Easter!

I remember visiting Grammy and Poppo's house during Christmas break and being surprised by snow (this was not a regular occurrence). Of course, nobody prepared for it, so we donned our tennis shoes wrapped in plastic trash bags and headed for some impromptu snow play! Christmas Eve was a huge event back at our house because my aunts and uncles would all come over and help my mom and dad set up the festive display from Santa under the tree. My uncles would spend hours and hours helping my dad, trying to get the slot cars (which required a significant amount of fine-tuning) ready to race before my brother awoke Christmas morning. Then there were the times when my cousins, sister, brother, and I would spend a week at "Camp Grammy and Poppo" (a much-anticipated event, I am sure, for our parents). One time, I, the oldest grandchild, had the fantastic idea that we would all "surprise" our grandparents by hiding out in the bathroom and cleaning it. Unfortunately, poor Grammy was beside herself when she couldn't find any of us.

We had a blast as we took many fun camping excursions to the beach with our extended family. Then, there was the time we had to "camp out" in our driveway for several days after we experienced the 1971 Sylmar 6.6 magnitude earthquake. Even though our house was severely damaged, I remember the excitement. My sister, brother, and I all sat on the two-seater swing in the backyard with our dog, Sammy, to protect us as my parents ensured that all the significant shaking had subsided and that the house was safe to re-enter. Our home, which was an older home built on concrete blocks, had sustained a considerable amount of damage. The water heater had flooded the kitchen and laundry room, and as we later explored the house, we found food inside the oven that had flown out of the fridge. We could even see my dad's shaving cream on the wall from his hasty exit. However, I must admit that my most terrifying concern was that my second-grade teacher, Mrs. Brown, would be mad because I wasn't in school that day. Mom assured me that even Mrs. Brown wouldn't be there! The adventure continued for many days until we could secure the house, make it safe to live in again, and eventually return to school.

These early years were eventful but full of mostly happy times. There were plenty of moments filled with fun, laughter, and the making of memories that would last a lifetime. Even though we may not have been financially well-off, we were rich in love for one another. Our family, both immediate and extended, was very close.

In the years to come, I would find out just how thankful I was for our family's togetherness and support. But unfortunately, those fond memories were soon eclipsed by new memories, which were not as joy-filled. Around the time I turned nine or ten, my life would drastically change. At first, it was very subtle, but it would soon affect my whole family. Gone would be the carefree years of childhood, and in their place would be over forty years of what would become an emotional and spiritual roller coaster.

CHAPTER TWO

# Change Is on the Horizon

My sister, Chrysty, was two years younger than me. She was a sweet, lovely girl with an infectious smile. An entry in my mother's journal beautifully describes her before and during her fight with Huntington's Disease.

*January 18, 1991*

*I remember her more and more as the sweet, smiling, impish young child. [My] memories of her as a young woman—beautiful, long flowing flaxen hair, a smile that could light the world of all those around her. [She had a] delightful sense of humor and, like her brother in later years of his life, [was] in a great deal of pain and confused...fighting for every minute of life available to her.*

———————————*(From the journal of Judith Bohlin)*

Chrysty and I were close to one another in our younger years, even dressing alike for Easter with outfits our mom had handcrafted. We loved playing together and doing what most elementary school-aged sisters do.

During her early school years, Chrysty started having difficulties with speech and other areas of learning.

*April 4, 1992* ———————————

*We fought to keep our daughter in regular education classes/schools as long as possible—she needed that exposure and challenge and thrived on it. When she did begin needing special help, the program that most closely fit her needs at that time was the Aphasia Program. It was not a perfect "fit" but the closest. [Unfortunately] it didn't last forever—her needs changed, and she transitioned into a program more suited to the physically/multi-handicapped.*

———————————*(From the journal of Judith Bohlin)*

Chrysty was placed in aphasia and learning disability classes to address some of her learning deficits. At first, no one was overly concerned and felt that she just needed some additional help. But, eventually, she started showing some signs of having difficulty with her balance and gait. After seeing various doctors and finally being referred to a neurologist, she was diagnosed with Huntington's Disease (HD). (Later we would come to see that she had actually been demonstrating signs of this disease as early as age three.) This disease is a dominantly inherited disorder, so doctors soon discovered that it was my father who carried the gene. In fact, unbeknownst to him, my mother, and his own family, Huntington's had existed on my father's side of the family for several generations. His father and grandfather likely had Huntington's but unfamiliarity with this disease at the time led to misdiagnoses of schizophrenia. They both eventually took their own lives. However, my father's symptoms were not overt, so they remained undetected. Likewise, Ronnie had not begun to show any signs either. So, while there would come a time when mom and I would be providing care for all three of our family's affected members, my sister primarily required the lion's share of our attention for most of my junior high and high school years.

*April 4, 1992*

*We didn't know such a thing as HD existed in our family or otherwise. Since we didn't, many of the early symptoms we had to cope with and had to try to figure out were very mysterious, perplexing, and confusing. The symptoms my children had were more identifiable before those eventually apparent in my husband. (He had changed, but unlike those of the children, they were assigned to other causes—stress, etc.). Because there was no family history, and because the symptoms looked so different in the children, their problems were not connected to those of their father until much later. (Our daughter began noticeable symptoms— change in gait and speech-slurring—at age 3; her brother at age 6 (same symptoms)—their father, at that time showing [signs,] but seemingly unrelated—was about 29 years of age).*

*(From the journal of Judith Bohlin)*

As I was close to Chrysty when we were younger, I tried to maintain involvement in her life even as her ability to interact with me declined. I began by volunteering in some of her special education classes (which would later spur me on to pursue a career in that field.) I also worked as a counselor at a camp for individuals with special needs for several years during high school and college. Both of my siblings attended that camp. At first, Chrysty was ambulatory, but as the years progressed, she became more physically involved and required constant care. By the time she was in her teens, she had to use a wheelchair, was bedridden, needed a feeding tube to continue eating, and could no longer communicate. Scheduling her appointments, care, and medications became a balancing act as we learned to navigate the storm created by Huntington's Disease.

*March 7, 1983*

*Chrysty was up and down again last night. My sleep again coming in one to two-hour bits. By 8:30 AM the phone was ringing—a friend, then the school; … another friend calling to offer to start filling 10 hours a week of the Homemaker-chore hours…Now staggering her 4-hour feeding schedule with med schedule, as she can't take ampicillin with food. Will try to lay down again for a few minutes before next feeding time as I have managed only 4-5 hours (in 24) sleep. Can't rest anyway as Chrysty is moaning & crying out—probably wet, so may as well get up. Changed Chrysty, fed her, cleaned & dressed tube site, gave bed bath. Enough for tonight. The time is now 1:20 AM, should be able to get her changed & fed by 1:40 AM—then maybe we can both rest. She should be tired, she's been awake almost continuously for 48 hours.*

———————————————*(From the journal of Judith Bohlin)*

CHAPTER THREE

# What's Happening to My Family?

My father, sister, and brother likely had a form of Juvenile Huntington's Disease (JHD). Interestingly, as noted below, the family history leading to the JHD form of Huntington's is often associated with the father, as was the case in both my father's family and our own.

---

Huntington's disease (HD) is a brain disease that is passed down in families from generation to generation. It is caused by a mistake in the DNA instructions that build our bodies and keep them running. DNA is made up of thousands of genes, and people with HD have a small error in one gene, called huntingtin. Over time this error causes damage to the brain and leads to HD symptoms.

HD causes deterioration in a person's physical, mental, and emotional abilities, usually during their prime working years, and currently has no cure. Most people start developing symptoms during adulthood, between the ages of 30 to 50, but HD can also occur in children and young adults (known as juvenile HD or JHD).[1]

---

---

*Juvenile Onset Huntington's Disease (JHD)* is a form of Huntington's disease (HD) that affects children and teenagers. Huntington's disease is a hereditary neurodegenerative disorder that is characterized by progressively worsening motor, cognitive, behavioral, and psychiatric symptoms. JHD is caused by a mutation of the huntingtin gene called a "CAG repeat expansion." The mutation results in gradual neuronal degeneration in the basal ganglia of the brain, which is responsible for coordination of movements, thoughts, and emotions. As JHD progresses, other regions of the brain undergo neuronal degeneration with diffuse and severe brain atrophy that is comparable to late stage *Alzheimer's disease.*

Predisposition and typical initial symptoms of Juvenile Onset HD include:

- Positive family history of HD, usually in the father
- Stiffness of the legs
- Clumsiness of arms and legs
- Decline in cognitive function
- Changes in behavior
- Seizures
- Changes in oral motor function
- Chorea in an adolescent
- Behavioral disturbances[2]

---

Huntington's Disease is rare, although I never knew just how rare until I began researching for this book. According to HDA.org.uk:

---

It is the same gene that determines whether you will develop Huntington's disease or Juvenile Huntington's disease. Everyone has it and it's called the Huntington's gene. It's found on chromosome pair number 4. However, people that develop either adult or Juvenile Huntington's have an important difference or 'fault' in their Huntington's gene...

If you have Juvenile or adult Huntington's disease, this means you inherited a faulty version of the Huntington's gene from one of your parents, and the recipe for the protein the gene produces is incorrect.

Less than 10% of people with the faulty Huntington's gene have more than 50 CAG repeats, making Juvenile Huntington's a very rare disease.

If you do have more than 50 repeats, there is a 90% chance you got the faulty gene from your father, as CAG repeats tend to be more unstable when passed on from the man. We don't yet know for sure why this is, but it is thought to be because the gene becomes more unstable in sperm.[3]

---

Over the next two decades, studies gained momentum, and in 1983 a marker carrying the gene was located. The Huntingtin (HTT) gene was the first disease-associated gene to be molecularly mapped to a human chromosome.[4] Ten years later, in 1993, the gene itself was found. These discoveries opened many doors for those at risk for the disease.

The rarity of Huntington's Disease and all it entailed in the 1970's added to the myriad of frustrations and caregiving concerns that my mother and I would face for the next 25 years.

CHAPTER FOUR

# Where it All Began

My father, Gerald, was a quiet man. While I cannot remember much about him during my early childhood, I know he was a loving father. One of my most cherished memories is my mother's story about a camera he gave me. Dad had saved who knows how many StarKist tuna labels to get me a camera shaped like Charlie the Tuna. I still have that camera. I love looking at photos of when he took me fishing, or allowed me to watch as he worked on his motorcycle. He never liked having his picture taken, as evidenced in most photos where he is holding up his hand in front of his face, but he was a handsome man, nonetheless. He was a carpenter and loved to work with his hands. To this day, I have a wooden bowl he crafted sitting in my kitchen as a memory of him. He specialized in door-hanging, but this became increasingly difficult for him and soon proved to be an indicator of his body's inability to function normally. His employers gradually gave him slightly easier tasks due to accidents and failure to complete his work. Eventually, by the time I reached my later elementary/junior high years, he could no longer work due to the disease's effects on his body and mind.

As mentioned previously, HD is a dominant-inherited disorder. After years of hearing a rudimentary backstory regarding my father's family, I gained a little more detail from Dad's sisters.

Dad and his siblings didn't know much about their grandfather (my great-grandfather) due to his early death by suicide. His father (my grandfather) was a family man who worked assorted jobs through the years to provide for his family. During a conversation with my Aunt Darlene, I gained some insight into what Dad had gone through as a young man; subsequently, I discovered that Huntington's Disease's presence in our family was, in all actuality, not such a surprise.

On one occasion, my aunt recalled their father getting mad about some sandwiches, literally out of the blue. He would yell and storm about and then, moments later, act as though nothing had happened.

In other instances, he would throw things, leave, and then call, saying he was lost. During these episodes, he never remembered what had happened. In addition to the memory loss, he also experienced muscle aches that doctors couldn't explain. In 1959, during a particularly violent fit of rage, he started hitting his wife, and my dad had to sit on him until he calmed down. Later that day, their father left home, never to return. He left a note addressed to my dad, which stated, "I can't handle the pain anymore or whatever is happening to me." My father, at eighteen, found him in the nearby river, having also committed suicide by drowning. As mentioned previously, it later became apparent that doctors had likely misdiagnosed Dad's grandfather and father as schizophrenic. In all likelihood, they were experiencing symptoms of Huntington's Disease, as would future generations.

Mom met my father in high school, and soon after graduation, they were married. Over the next eight years, they had three children, not knowing that my father had Huntington's Disease and thus a 50% chance of transmitting it to his children.

This devastating disease passed on by my grandfather and great-grandfather would soon be brought to light through the disease diagnosis in my sister, Chrysty, and subsequently, in my brother, Ronnie. My father had unknowingly passed the gene onto another generation.

*April 4, 1992* ———

*By the time our son began showing symptoms—he was the second in line to show changes—we did begin to suspect the connection between the two and that what was happening to them appeared progressive. I can remember the dread, the horror. I remember the doctors ruling out various possibilities. With ruling out one, I would be so relieved, as though I were at top of a very long hard climb only to be told that the other remaining possibilities, each time, were even worse—the plummet from the top to the bottom, a real roller coaster ride. Finally, their symptoms were linked to their father's now more apparent symptoms and I was told that, in all probability they all three had a progressive, terminal illness; one that really embodied the worst parts of all the others which had been previous possibilities. Little did I ever dream that the time would come when I would have given anything for my husband and children to have had one of those [other] maladies because, at least, for most of them there was some knowledge, some treatment. I was told, for HD there was no treatment and very little was known about it, and that our eldest, was at risk for the disease as well!*

——————————————(*From the journal of Judith Bohlin*)

In retrospect, my mom began to understand those first subtle changes that had been taking place in her husband while they were dating. During high school, he had been an avid ice skater and a good student. Yet, when they were dating, his grades suddenly worsened, and he quit ice skating for no apparent reason. Most likely, this was due to the changes that were taking place in his body's ability to balance; and in his mind's ability to learn and retain knowledge. But, as I said, these changes were so subtle at first that no one thought twice about them. Given that Huntington's Disease was not a well-known, researched, or discussed disorder in the medical community back in the late 1950's and '60s, it is no wonder that it had gone unnoticed for multiple generations; and would now continue to leave its mark on those in the future.

CHAPTER FIVE

# The Relentless Battle

During the latter years of Chrysty's life, my father's and brother's symptoms worsened. The dementia aspect of Huntington's Disease took its toll on Dad. He gradually became confused and, at times, aggressive, just as his father had been. I recall times when Mom was attempting to go somewhere, and he would want to go along with her. When this was not a possibility, she would try to explain why he could not accompany her, and then he would be left in my care. In one of my diary entries, I mentioned one incident when he was attempting to chase after her car, and I was trying to stop him. He wouldn't respond and fought against my efforts. Eventually, my mother had to return and intervene. I "ran to my room and cried." Other times, chasing after the car caused him to fall and injure himself.

On one occasion, a friend found him on the main boulevard nearby. Such incidents became normative for Mom and me.

Eventually, Dad's behavior became too aggressive and difficult for us to manage. We had placed many calls to 911 where the police and psych units would come to our home, but by the time they arrived, he was calm, so there was nothing they could do to help.

I remember the day, in 1983, when he was removed from our home. For some reason, he was upset and trying to gain access to my mom, who had locked herself in their bedroom. He was trying to get the door off the hinges (having been a door-hanger gave him the knowledge of how to do this). Mom called out to me from behind the locked door, and told me to take Ronnie and the phone and lock ourselves in the bathroom. She told me to call 911 and tell them what was happening. Chrysty was bedridden at this point, and we were confident that he would not try to harm her, so she remained in her room. There had been incidences, though, when my dad would get overly physical with Ronnie, so I assume that is why she had us lock ourselves safely in the bathroom. It was not an easy call to make that day. The police and a psych response team arrived, and this time he was still agitated to the point that they felt it was best to remove him from our home. He would never return.

After being admitted to a psychiatric ward at the nearby hospital, he progressively worsened. The doctors treated him as a psychological patient, not a Huntington's Disease patient with psychological problems. This distinction made a big difference in his care and medical attention. They administered medications usually given to psychological patients, such as those with schizophrenia. These drugs were of the phenothiazine type, and a major one used was Thorazine. My mother discovered that this family of treatments can have a "paradoxical" action or even worsen some of the choreic movements associated with Huntington's Disease. As a result of this mistake, my dad suffered a significant amount of physical illness and neared a pneumonic state. Fortunately, Mom was able to get him transferred to a different hospital before any further deterioration occurred. One of the outcomes of this initial placement, and subsequent effects on his body, was confinement to a wheelchair (upon entering the original institution, he had been ambulatory.)

*March 20, 1983*

*Almost two weeks have passed since I last wrote. It seems like two months at least! We did have to take Gerald to be seen and evaluated by the Director of Nurses at the possible [new] placement—who refused to see him after the long trip over there. The administrator immediately asked Gerald if this was where he wanted to live, which, of course, gave Gerald the idea he had a choice and, naturally, his choice would be to live at home. Obviously, since "home" wasn't one of his choices, it could only go downhill from that point; each time the question was asked (and it was repeated many more times coming from the misplaced, misguided intentions of the administrator of a locked facility), yet it only served to reinforce Gerald's resolve to refuse to live anywhere but home, since he now supposedly had a choice! He ended up trying to leave Magnolia Gardens [a placement that occurred after the initial psych hospital visit upon removal from our home] that evening and several times the next day to come "home" and got combative when they tried to physically restrain him. So, by the next day (actually by 8:30 AM) I received my first call of the day informing me that the facility was calling an ambulance to have Gerald transferred [back] to county psych hospital and that I needed to come immediately with conservatorship papers to affect the transfer. I was not surprised having witnessed the sight of his having to be held by a male nurse and two other staff to keep him from following my car. The next few days have gotten worse by the day.*

———————————*(From the journal of Judith Bohlin)*

At this point, I started to appreciate just how vital my extended family had been and would continue to be, in our lives, especially mine. They attended doctor's appointments, assisted with care, and offered emotional support to our family.

So many years later, I would come to understand what a treasured gift God had given me in the form of my grandparents and many uncles, aunts, and cousins. They provided a much-needed "normalcy" in my life. For example, my uncles ensured I always had a working car to drive to college, and helped pay for books and other necessities. They also built a hope chest for me as I looked forward to life one day outside my home. One of my aunts took me on camping excursions for respite. My family even sent me on a Hawaiian vacation after my college graduation. We remain very close to one another to this day. Their support was so important then and would prove even more crucial later in my life.

As my mother and I continued to fight what seemed to be an ongoing uphill battle regarding caregiving and advocating for those in our family affected by HD, I don't think I ever knew the magnitude of what Mom went through.

*March 20, 1983*

*Gathered necessary papers (formidable number)—Dad offered to go along for moral support and mom stayed to oversee Chrysty's care as a friend hadn't arrived. When we arrived at the county hospital, Gerald waited rather nervously to see the doctor. They were replacing some seating and kept asking Gerald, who was very apprehensive by this time, to move. Then the doctor came to take him into a "holding area"— a large room where everyone was restrained to a bed—beds with agitated people everywhere—some chanting, some cursing, some screaming, some crying. Gerald remembered the place from his first visit when he was initially taken from home. He kept saying, "Please don't let them tie me down!" He became very frightened and combative (resistive). They wouldn't allow either of us to go with Gerald to calm or reassure him.*

*[Mom goes on to share how he got upset about his ring being taken and how they said he had to sign*

*a waiver to keep it. Then, finally, a guard realized how vital...]*

*...that one last link with reality and security was to Gerald and returned it to him immediately. Everyone must be treated as the least reachable case and as sub-human. As a reasonably sane person, this is how I saw the happenings of that day—imagine how frightening it must have been to those having a tenuous hold on reality already but [who were] still feeling people—such as Gerald.*

———————————*(From the journal of Judith Bohlin)*

In other journal entries, my mother said she signed paperwork without being told what it addressed. After asking questions before signing other papers, she finally found out it was for permission to transfer my father to a psych ward at a state hospital. After many calls had been made and new medications for behavior control were administered, they were able to move him back to a regular hospital. As a result of the numerous occasions dealing with doctors regarding the nuances of Huntington's and the outbursts associated with the dementia aspect of it, she began to see a pattern. The meds used to control the behavior and outbursts were causing increased agitation instead. He became medically unstable and had bruises that showed the deterioration that had taken place.

Unfortunately, many homes and facilities during the 1980s were not equipped for, nor did they have trained staff to deal with someone who had Huntington's Disease. Dad began to wander from the unlocked facility he was residing in and was repeatedly found walking down crowded boulevards. It became evident that this was not a safe place for him. In 1983, Mom decided to have him placed at Fairview State Hospital, where he remained for the next thirteen years, until he died in 1996 at the age of fifty-five.

CHAPTER SIX

# The First Loss

The year 1983 continued to be a challenging and devastating one for me. Not only was my father removed from our home, but I also came to realize that the days of carefree sisterly play were long gone and would never return. Chrysty's care was very involved, so I became one of her regular caregivers whenever Mom needed a break or had a meeting to attend. She was bedridden and now had a feeding tube that required special training to administer food.

Eventually, the constant seizures took their toll on my sister's body, and on October 22, 1983, at the age of seventeen, Chrysty passed away while still at our home.

I was in my second year at Cal State University, Northridge, but still living at home and helping to care for my sister. I remember that night vividly. Mom was away at a much-needed retreat (which was not usually an option for her), and a few friends from the summer camp I worked at were over for a visit. As I proceeded to brief the night nurse on the last feeding times/medications, etc., we headed toward my sister's room. We found her lying there in the bed, not breathing. The nurse administered CPR but to no avail. Chrysty had quietly passed away. The doctor later explained that the part of her brain that told her body to breathe had ceased functioning. I remember being simultaneously upset and relieved that I, not my mom, had found her. (This is just one example of how Mom and I tried to protect one another.)

It wasn't until a few years later (I believe as the Lord was working on my heart and drawing me closer to Him) that I would stop to think about some of the feelings regarding the loss of my sister that night and how they had affected me.

Taken from a therapy session letter I wrote "to my sister" after her death:

> *I don't want to die. [I'm] afraid of dying myself [and] of going to sleep and not waking up like Chrysty did. She couldn't breathe—and I'm afraid I won't be able to breathe—felt really bad when Chrysty died like it was*

*my fault. I had caused her to stop breathing by not checking on her. She couldn't breathe, but I have been reassured by Mom that the reason Chrysty couldn't breathe was because she had nothing telling her to breathe inside her brain.*

*Chrysty—I'm not sorry you died when you did—but only because I didn't want to have to see you go through any more pain. I didn't want anyone else to either. I hope you can forgive me for wanting you to die—but it wasn't you that I wanted to die—it was the HD—just the same as it is with Ron and Dad. If I could have had a sister without HD; or if we could have just grown up together sharing a little bit more of our normal lives together; or if we could have been both normal—I wouldn't have wanted a sister any other than you—I only wish that there was more of our lives together that we might have been able to talk with each other as sisters do, that I could remember. I really miss remembering the good part of our lives together when we were little kids and when HD hadn't really affected you or the family very much—because if I could remember that part of our lives I'd have something to remember that was really good and happy. I do remember from pictures when Mom made us those matching dresses for Easter. I wish there were some way of us talking now. I can't say that I wish I would have been in your place—but I definitely have lived thinking about being at risk. I've also tried to go on and live as normal of a life as I can. Maybe it's for both of us. Maybe I will go on living my life for both of us.*

*I really wish you didn't have to be alone—and to tell you the truth, I can't remember if I told you I love you before I left the room—I also don't know if I could have stayed in the room w/ you as you were dying—and I hope you know that in my heart, I really wish I could have. I hope that you can forgive me for not being there and for maybe not wanting to be there, and I hope you don't hate me for it. Although, as nice a sister as I remember you being—and as I could have hoped for—I don't think you will have hated me. I hope your dying when you did, and how you did, was just your way of finally letting go. I hope that if there was any way of you living any meaningful life at the point you were at, you would have gone on living it. I just hope you know that I will always remember you. If I could have been strong enough to be in your room holding your hand and telling you I love you I hope you know I would have been. I hope you know that I only hated the disease and not you, and that if there were any way to separate the two, I would have. I'm sorry that you had to die without any of us nearby or talking with you—but I hope that my brief few moments in the room [earlier] were enough to let you know we were there. I just hope you know that I love you and that I would have been there if there were any way I could have been with you.*

*I love you the mostest, Chrysty.*

*Love,*
*Your sister, Lyndy*

CHAPTER SEVEN

# Time Marches On

Chrysty's death left a massive hole in our hearts, but the demands of caregiving and living with the effects of Huntington's Disease relentlessly continued. In addition to my father's removal and subsequent placement in a state hospital and my sister's death, Ronnie, now sixteen, began to worsen. However, it seemed he had remained ambulatory and more capable for longer than my sister.

*November 14, 1983*

*Ronnie had his first seizure on Saturday, Nov. 12, 1983. I can't believe that it happened. This seems like a nightmare that I haven't awakened from. It doesn't seem fair to him, or to anyone else. Poor Mom hasn't had any break. Now she has to start the cycle all over again. I hope for Ronnie's sake that he doesn't have to go through all the suffering Chrysty did. Things are getting harder to handle instead of easier. School is getting rough [for me]—so many exams. Finals are in 4 weeks! I hope I can keep up the strength to make it through the semester. I hate to have wasted all this time.*

———*From my journal*

Ronnie was the youngest child in our family. He was quite the jokester, generally outgoing, and even had a girlfriend for many years. Despite our age differences, he and I developed more of a "sibling bond." I volunteered at his school and even rode the bus with him on occasion while I was finishing my training as a special education teacher. We celebrated our junior high and high school graduations together. He and I talked about things my sister and I had not been able to discuss and his awareness and capability to understand what was happening to him were more apparent than Chrysty's. After all, he had seen, firsthand, what she experienced.

I recall the day we were locked together in the bathroom (away from Dad). We were awaiting the arrival of the emergency personnel, and Ronnie asked me whether he was going to wind up like our sister—bedridden in the room next door. I can't recall how I responded, but I know it wasn't an easy discussion.

At a young age, Ronnie's peers made fun of the rigidity of his body. His transition to a special education campus provided an opportunity for him to thrive. No one called him "robot man," and the staff and students loved him as he was an integral part of the community there.

Throughout my college years, my brother and I spent time together in ways Chrysty and I never did. With the help of others, we attended special events like a Jackson 5 concert and a Dodger baseball game that a college friend had arranged. It was particularly memorable for my brother because the team signed a baseball just for him. Thanks to the Make-A-Wish Foundation, we were fortunate enough to visit Florida, along with my future stepdad and my mom. The four of us visited both Disney World and Cypress Gardens. It was a trip I would never forget and a pleasant memory amidst the sadness that so often surrounded our family.

I feel as though we were a little more "prepared" when it came to providing care for my brother. Despite HD's effects on his body, he didn't seem to succumb as rapidly or as devastatingly as my sister did at first. Ronnie lived to be twenty-one years-old, and for most of his life, we had been able to care for him in our home. However, despite our best efforts, he required occasional hospitalization to adjust his medications. Unfortunately, during one of these visits, they found that Ronnie's hip was broken. Instead of repairing it, they decided that since he was no longer ambulatory, the best course of action was to cut his leg tendons. While he was in the hospital recovering from that surgery, he became septic. On February 26, 1990, just a short time after I had become engaged to be married, Ronnie passed away.

During his funeral, the outpouring of love and support was overwhelming. Many counselors he and I knew from our years at Camp Joan Mier came that day. Without exaggerating, I can say that half of the staff from the special education school he attended and the one I currently worked at filled the church. So many were present that day that those two schools were short-staffed. I can see now that these people were part of the growing group of individuals that God used to help Mom and me make it through some of the most challenging moments in our lives. Essentially, they provided some much-needed light in the darkness of our grief as Huntington's Disease continued to cast a shadow on our lives.

CHAPTER EIGHT

# Will it Ever End?

Huntington's Disease seemed all-consuming for much of my life, between caring for affected family members and being at risk for the same life-altering disease. While Mom and I experienced many of the same emotions and difficulties adjusting to life with HD in our family, I know we had differing viewpoints and each employed different coping mechanisms. She was, after all, a mother and wife, while I was a sister, daughter, and the only remaining family member to be at-risk for HD. So not only did my mom have to deal with the heartache associated with the required daily care provided, but she also carried great concern about what kind of life I would have if I also tested positive for the gene.

*November 16, 1990*

*When Jerry...dies,...HD and a family with affected members will end. Lyndy will either not be at risk, or will most likely have the gene—depending upon the outcome of the test, causing the HD in the family to play a role dependent upon that outcome. Whatever that outcome, though some will begin to feel otherwise, we will always be an HD family—either a family who had, or a family who has HD.*

*(From the journal of Judith Bohlin)*

Mom chose to deal with her challenges by arming herself with knowledge and training, but my reaction and subsequent actions weren't so directed. Instead, I think I often operated on autopilot, which sometimes worked but didn't always provide a safe landing.

I was still in elementary school when I first encountered and began understanding the magnitude of Huntington's Disease and how it would affect my life. I know I had started to question why my sister, and sometimes my father, had different physical movements and capabilities than my friends' family members. For the most part, I think I primarily relied on my mother's strength and example and was naïve regarding its seriousness. Life had not changed too drastically, so as far as I was concerned, things were still reasonably normal.

By the time I entered junior high, I had begun to understand that things would not get better regarding our family situation. I realized that this illness would not one day go away, and my sister, brother, and father were all getting worse. Finances were tight, and now there were more people in my life with whom I interacted, who knew about HD in our family. Some friends knew I had a "handicapped" sister who required care. However, I don't think they questioned much about Dad's or Ronnie's actions yet, and likely just dismissed them as being shy or reclusive. I know I must have understood that I was at risk for HD by this point in my life, but I don't recall dwelling on it much.

The reality of being at risk for HD hit home during my high school years. By this point, I was aware that I had a 50-50 chance of inheriting the same faulty gene that my father, sister, brother, and likely grandfather and great-grandfather had all received. As a result, I started attending more support groups with Mom as the years went by. It was there that I encountered others who were also at risk.

I recall being conflicted about attending these group meetings because I had to acknowledge the reality of Huntington's Disease in my family and the possibility that I might be a carrier. Sometimes it was nice to speak to a kindred spirit who might be experiencing the same emotions I was, but most of the time, I did not enjoy talking with them at length because it reminded me of the daily fate with which I now struggled.

The many demands for my attention often relegated concern over being at risk to a back burner. Instead, I found myself striving to live a "normal" life as a young adolescent and later as an adult woman, despite the caregiving burdens I faced. I participated in marching band and attended football games. I excelled in my studies and pursued scholarships. I even tried out for cheerleading my senior year and went to the prom. During the year, I worked at a bookstore and in the summer at a camp for the disabled. After graduating with honors, I headed for California State University, Northridge, where I pursued my bachelor's degree in Liberal Studies, two teaching credentials, and a master's degree in special education. I was busy focusing on my studies, working to pay for school, and caring for family members with HD. I became more involved in the Los Angeles Chapter of Huntington's Disease Society alongside Mom and attended national conferences. Yet, despite my juggling prowess, when it came to this stage of my life, "living with HD" still affected me.

I had tried to be there to help Mom as much as I could. After all, it was just she and I, for the most part, who were responsible for most of the care associated with the three other members of our five-person family. Throughout the disease process, that care varied depending on which stage of the disease each was experiencing. Yet, while I continued to support my mom with the daily assistance my sister, brother, and father required, I fought a silent battle within, wondering if one day I, too, would need that very same care.

I like to think I was strong and resilient, but I know it took its toll. Physically, my anxiety became apparent in the form of trichotillomania—hair pulling as a way of dealing with stress and anxiety (although I did not figure out the connection until my college years when I had to write a report about it). It seemed that, no matter how hard I tried, the fear and anxiety of being at risk for HD were just as present in my life now as they had been before.

For over 25 years of my life, I wondered if, worried about, and sometimes even assumed that HD would soon manifest itself within my mind and body. Part of me was concerned that I, too, would just lie down to go to sleep one night and stop breathing as my sister had.

I recall times when, if I stumbled or fell, I would immediately begin to question whether it was the beginning signs of the same wretched disease. All the support groups, therapists, and even Mom, couldn't remove the overwhelming feeling that I was carrying the Huntington's Disease gene.

I think a lot of the emotional aspects of what I had been dealing with started to come to a head on that night Chrysty passed away. For many years, no matter how hard I tried to move on, I still could not entirely absolve myself of the feeling that I had somehow allowed her to die that night.

Even as I write this over 39 years later, I am still moved to tears as I think back on that evening. I struggled with Chrysty's death. I mourned the loss of the sister that I, in some ways, never really had. Guilt plagued me on many different levels. I felt like I had somehow caused her death. I experienced guilt over the relief I felt that she had died. I suppose I even felt remorse that I, so far, had managed to escape the disease that had ravaged her body. Upon recommendations from a counselor, I wrote that note to my sister expressing all my guilt. I suppose it was a means to get me to see that it wasn't my desire for her to die. Instead, it was the HD within her that I was glad was gone.

Guilt was not a new emotion to me. Throughout the years of driving back and forth from the San Fernando Valley to Costa Mesa, where my father would reside in the state hospital for the rest of his life, I experienced a lot of guilt and even anger. As a teenager, I was pretty distraught at holidays because we would almost always miss out on the "big" family celebration at Grammy and Poppo's by the time we had made our way back through holiday traffic from visiting Dad. It was also tricky having a father in a state hospital and siblings at home, both of whom required constant care and assistance and could not be left alone. I felt guilt over the resentment I carried toward the loss of a "normal," everyday life, both for myself and my family.

As I have looked back at my life during those years of being a caregiver, while I was also at risk for the same disease that would eventually take three members of our family, I know now that God gave me glimpses of His love for me. Those glimpses enabled me to survive all the emotional ups and downs, including the anxiety, guilt, and sadness. I just did not realize it until later.

CHAPTER NINE

# My New Normal

Life continued despite the behind-the-scenes drama that often occupied my days. After completing my bachelor's degree, I began working on the two teaching credentials. Near the end of the process, I had to finish my student teaching. During this time, I was still living at home and working at the summer camp. Upon completing my student teaching I applied to work as a substitute teacher while interviewing for a full-time position. During that summer of 1985, my life would take yet another turn.

Ever since I was a child, I had believed in God's existence. I went to Sunday school and church with my family. I tried my best to be a "good girl." As far as I was concerned, I was doing a great job. In addition to being a caregiver, I was still working hard at being involved in school and getting good grades, and I had a plan to succeed in life. This plan would not be dictated by the various concerns and responsibilities associated with Huntington's Disease. I went to college, stayed away from drugs, was in and out of bad relationships, and partied a little here and there, but I figured I was still on good terms with God because I had not murdered anyone or stolen anything. After all, *those* were sins. With all the emotional turmoil of losing a sister and continuing to care for other family members afflicted by HD, I occasionally felt a need to talk to God. However, most of the time, I figured I was doing fine all on my own.

Then one day, I had an unexpected weird, isolated seizure incident. While driving on the freeway, I blacked out and miraculously ended up parked on a nearby street corner with a flat tire and no recollection of how I got there. Doctors attributed it to psychosomatic seizure syndrome (basically, they could not determine the exact cause, although stress and heat-related issues were possible factors). I remember lying there in the doctor's office that day. I must have thought my life was ending because I started confessing to Mom what I then realized was questionable behavior, especially over the past few years in college. When it was clear that I wasn't going to die at that moment, I started worrying that this could be the beginning signs of the dreaded Huntington's since my afflicted family members all had seizures. I am sure that Mom had those very same concerns. However, the neurologist caring for the members of my family with HD assured me this incident was not associated. I did feel some relief after his reassurances, but it was still a wake-up call regarding how I had been living my life in general. It was during this time that I began to change. I started to sense a need for dependence on Someone other than myself.

I was unable to drive for almost a year until they were sure I wouldn't have any more seizures. As I navigated this new temporary reality, I had to rely on transportation from friends, Mom, or even riding the school bus alongside my brother to continue my student teaching and subsequent substitute teaching assignments. Eventually, I returned to driving and secured a long-term position at a local special education school, which later became a full-time assignment. I moved out of my family home and began living independently for the first time. I met a fellow school employee and his friend, who invited me to come to a young adult group at their church. The funny thing was this church was back in the same neighborhood where I had spent my childhood! It was these same two friends who, months later, shared the gospel with me. I now understood that just believing in God's existence and occasionally checking in with Him was not enough. Just knowing *of* Him was not the same as *knowing* Him. I needed to have a personal relationship with Him. This relationship required that I trust that He was, and always will be, Who He says He is. I needed to accept His grace, forgiveness, love, strength, and most of all, His gift of His one and only Son, Jesus Christ, as my Lord, Creator, and personal Savior. It wasn't an earth-shattering moment or filled with any lightning strike, but that day, in January of 1989, Jesus forever changed my heart.

Since that day, it saddens me to think that it took me almost 27 years to find Jesus. Then God reminded me that even though I didn't acknowledge my need for Him during those first 27 years, He had still been there. He started bringing to mind many instances throughout my life where He had been there. For example, God had led me to my friend at work, who later shared the gospel with me. He even orchestrated my life so that the skills I learned in caring for my family members would enable me to succeed in the field of special education and thus ultimately meet the man of my dreams. Therefore, instead of feeling sad due to years of not walking in a relationship with Him, I am praising Him for never leaving my side.

God showed me ways that His presence brought joy amidst the sorrow. I recalled a day when we were visiting Dad, and out of the blue, he had a few moments where he talked with me. It was something he had not been able to do for several years. It passed so quickly that I was almost unsure whether it had occurred, yet I now know it was God's way of giving me glimpses of my earthly Dad that I longed to know.

He reminded me of the many provisions that had sustained me throughout the years. One such example was my extended family, who provided things Mom could not: a car (including maintenance and repairs on it for many years), financial help with college, and that cherished trip for my college graduation. My family loved me and my sister, brother, and father as if HD did not exist. My dad's side of the family (who lived outside of the state) had also reached out from afar and supported us. They provided opportunities for me to get away and visit. They also did their best to come to California and see us as often as possible. There were so many other things that may not have meant much to me at the time that I later came to appreciate. For example, my pediatrician gave my mother the money to purchase a prom dress so I could attend my senior prom and charged discounted rates when we had to visit him. Youth group leaders and next-door neighbors stepped in, sometimes in the spur of the moment, providing necessary care for my siblings. There were friends from the camp who remained close, giving me much-needed support during some difficult times, and several friends from school who went with me to visit my dad or take my brother on excursions. Most importantly, He gave me a mother determined to help me experience a somewhat "normal" life. I can see how she exhibited selfless acts of love, commitment, and strength that God knew I needed back then and would continue to build upon as I began my independent life.

---

> We sing because we see God. We see his might and are reminded of his love. We remember that he has always come through for us and that his mercy has never failed us.[5]
>
> —*Louie Giglio*

I am now learning to be thankful for how His strength was always there for me despite the hardships in my childhood. First, I had Mom, my earthly example, rock, and anchor. Then later, my husband and sons would become my support system as I would soon enter into the next season of life with its hardships. I learned that He will always be there for me—molding and strengthening me. There would continue to be moments of strength, faith, and, yes, even times of weakness and doubt. But I started to become more confident in my knowledge that He has, is, and always will be the constant, never-changing Lord of my life. As a result of that newfound knowledge, I desire to live my life so that I will be filled with more of Him and less of me. Fear and anxiety continue to rear their ugly heads, but now I have an unwavering strength that I can rely on instead of my own. How I would weather the next storm that came my way would be drastically different.

> *My salvation and my honor depend on God; he is my mighty rock, my refuge.*
>
> *Trust in him at all times, you people; pour out your hearts to him, for God is our refuge.*
>
> *Psalm 62:7–8*

CHAPTER TEN

# The Wonder Years

I secured a full-time position in the Autistic department at the special education school, where I had worked as a sub. My class was comprised of seven students, most of whom were younger men taller and stronger than me, but I was excited to have this new job. There were four teachers in the department: three girls and one guy, and we were a close-knit group. Well, at least the girls were. We supported one another when dealing with students and even went on field trips together. I loved my new job and enjoyed the camaraderie we shared. Outside work, I was having fun attending the young adult gatherings at my new church and did not desire to spend my life partying at local clubs as I previously had. In addition, I was no longer in the long-term relationship I had been in for the past three years and didn't date much, so it was nice to have new friends.

I was growing in my faith and excited about life in general. I now had a place of my own, a full-time teaching position, and even a new car. I continued to assist with my brother's care by offering respite when Mom needed it or couldn't get help. She continued advocating on behalf of HD patients by conducting in-services at various group homes, leading support groups, testifying at multiple hearings, and raising awareness for the need to advance the research to locate the elusive Huntington's gene and subsequent cure. In addition to all of this, she remained active in the local organization. I increased my participation in the Los Angeles chapter by producing the newsletter and acting as the Board Secretary. However, while HD was still a big part of my life, I sought to make it "my" life instead of a life dictated by HD.

In January of 1989, several of us from work decided to go skiing at Mammoth, a ski resort in Northeast California. Even though I had problems with my rental skis several times during the day, it was still a great excursion. As the afternoon progressed, it began to snow heavily, so we ended our time with one more trip down the mountain. Unfortunately, it was during that last run of the day that my accident happened. My ski planted in the fresh snow, and the binding on the rental boots that I had struggled with all day long didn't release. My momentum carried the rest of me forward while my left leg remained stuck in the snow, so I fell, broke my tibia, and tore the surrounding ligaments. After being transported by ambulance to the local hospital, they determined I would need surgery to repair the damage by reattaching it all with a screw. All my friends eventually returned home, but I stayed behind for several days so that they could monitor my progress. Even though I felt alone, I knew I wasn't. It was one of the first occasions I had to test my newfound faith in God. As I lay there looking out a window blocked by snow with my leg hooked up to a machine that moved it imperceptibly to decrease stiffening, I took heart in the fact that I was going to be okay. I had my Bible to keep me company, and I could talk with God. I sensed His care for me and knew He was watching over me. This newfound communication with God and sense of His presence were welcomed changes in my life. After three days in the hospital, the surgeon flew me home on his private jet, and I headed to Mom's house to recuperate. But recuperation wasn't the only healing I was going to experience. Soon, I would know an overwhelming sense of restoration and rebirth.

Let me rewind my story a little—for clarity. As I mentioned before, I had been in and out of various dating relationships during my early adult years. I can see now how God was protecting me during that time. They weren't all bad, but I know that some of the types of guys I dated were likely my way of not fully acknowledging my underlying concern that I was not "long-term or marriage" material because I was at risk for Huntington's Disease. I think a not-so-small voice in my head told me that to consider marrying me would mean that you had to accept "tainted goods." So, I dated some men who were more into what was in it for them rather than pursuing a relationship with me. Yet, after accepting Christ and understanding the depth of God's love for me, I could see He loved me no matter what. He had created me to be the person I was. It didn't matter if I had Huntington's Disease. He would give me the strength to get through dealing with all that entailed. I saw the necessity of focusing on Him and living my life in such a way that I trusted His sovereignty over it all. I needed to date someone who loved God, saw me as He did, and cared more for me than themselves.

The secretaries in the front office at my school were these sweet older ladies who were aspiring matchmakers. On occasion, they would suggest that the "one guy" from the Autistic department and I go on a date together. At first, we saw it as a silly notion, but given their unrelenting attempts to see it come to fruition, we finally conceded and decided to go out, just once. We agreed upon a date, but it subsequently happened to fall during the week after my skiing accident. Upon my return home from the hospital, Rob (that guy) called me to ask if we were still on for our obligatory date. I explained that I was residing at my mom's home until I could navigate the stairs at my condo. Much to my surprise, he offered to bring dinner and a movie to Mom's so we could still have our "date." As we sat and enjoyed our BBQ dinner from a local restaurant called Love's and watched an old comedy called "Love at First Bite," we jointly decided that perhaps we should go out on an actual date because, after all, this didn't count. (To this day, I still tease about his food and movie choices on that first date.)

We went out on that second date a week later, and the quiet dinner at a nice restaurant allowed us to get to know one another. At that point, I decided to tell Rob I was at risk for Huntington's Disease. In retrospect, I feel that a part of me thought he would smile, enjoy the time together that night, and then never call again. But, months later, I would understand and come to cherish this man's heart and love for me.

Rob did call again. And again. We started to date a few months later exclusively, and by January of the following year, he proposed. Rob told me that the commitment he saw to my family, as exhibited by my mother, and myself, was one of the traits he most admired about me. His love for my family (which consisted of my mom, brother, and father at this point) exceeded any I could imagine. But even more remarkable was his love for Jesus and me. I saw this evidenced by his agreement to marry me even though I might carry the Huntington's Disease gene. He trusted God's sovereignty enough to enter our marriage with eyes wide open, and this is one of the biggest blessings I feel God has ever given me. However, mixed with the joy associated with my upcoming marriage was sorrow. Shortly after Rob proposed, my brother, Ronnie, passed away. His death brought back the intense grief I had lived through a few years earlier with my sister's passing, but this time I felt more peace as I dealt with the sorrow. God had not only given me my mother, friends, and family to lean on, but He had also given me Rob. The strength from Rob and the peace that only God can provide enabled me to get through this second loss.

In April of 1990, Rob and I were married and thus began the next season of my life. We were fortunate to find a new home within a few months and started our lives as husband and wife. We had discussed our desire to have children but agreed that we would wait until I could go through testing for HD. After locating the marker carrying the Huntington's Disease gene, predictive testing was nearly available, and I would later become one of the first people in Southern California to be tested. Unfortunately, it was not something that could give you a definitive yes or no result (as the later gene test would provide); however, this test could tell you somewhere between 50-99.9% whether you carried the gene. Given my family history and the blood from affected and unaffected family members, my mother had diligently "banked," I could proceed with testing that would later provide results with a high level of accuracy. Rob and I began the process of waiting for those results. It took months of counseling and testing, but we received the anticipated phone call later that year. I will never forget that day. The doctor called me at work, and the principal instructed the secretary to put the call through to my room, knowing that it was the long-awaited results. He said I was not a carrier of the HD gene based on my family history, bloodwork, and test results. I quickly ran down the hall to Rob's room to give him the news and promptly called my mom.

*March 1991*

*Lyndy is 98%+ free of markers that travel with the HD gene! Such an incredible revelation! The news was so overwhelming. She seems like (she is, in many ways) a different person. It is hard to realize that for us, with her father's death, HD will be over...(for our immediate family.) Having lived for so many years with acceptance of the idea that Lyndy is at-risk and either would have no children, or would adopt, or would have a child at-risk—It's a foreign feeling to know she is not at risk and that she can have a child with no more risk than anyone.*

*(From the journal of Judith Bohlin)*

She summed it up nicely. It was a "foreign feeling" to think I would be able to move on with my life and actively pursue having a family. Yet, in my ongoing list of abundant blessings from the Lord, I was praising Him for the opportunity I had previously thought was entirely unattainable. For many of my latter adult years, I had lived my life in such a way that I didn't allow myself to think about the possibility of marriage, let alone children.

Having received the good news stating that I did not carry the Huntington's gene, Rob and I decided to begin trying to start a family. Later that year, we were blessed by the birth of our first son. Over the next four years, we welcomed two more sons, and our little family was now a family of five. We continued to visit my father in the state hospital during that time. Rob, Mom, and I remained active in the Los Angeles Chapter of the Huntington's Disease Society. The Lord even allowed my dad to live long enough that all three of our young sons were able to meet him. Unfortunately, in October of 1996, he passed away. His last few months were rough and he was in hospice care. As difficult as it was to be there with him in the last hours, I think God had enabled me to grieve slowly over the years. During all the time he was in placement, I had begun to say goodbye. With his death, the prevalence of 25 years of Huntington's Disease no longer existed in our little family.

During the 1990s, my faith grew. Not only did I no longer have the shroud of Huntington's Disease hanging over my life, but I was also now a wife and mother. I came to understand these roles through the lens of His Word. I can say that the most extensive growth probably came during our homeschooling years, as my love, joy, peace, patience, kindness, goodness, faithfulness, gentleness, and self-control were *all* tested at length. Throughout those years, I was humbled in many ways as a wife and mother. I learned to respect Rob's position as the spiritual leader in our home and sought to grow in my role in raising our sons in a godly way. I remember crying out to Him in frustration as I tried to fulfill my duties and follow the path He set out before me. He continued to show me His presence and ongoing forgiveness even during moments of failure; and His love for me as I sought to honor Him.

Yes, I had grown in my faith and trust in the Lord. I could readily see His blessings and His hand in my life. Yet, as I would soon understand, I was still operating considerably in my strength. I sought to follow God, obey Him, and honor Him but was still often doing so on my terms. As I embarked on this next voyage across the stormy seas of my life, I learned I needed to surrender fully and allow His strength to work in me.

CHAPTER ELEVEN

# The Struggle Was Real

My mom, Judith, was a strong woman who fought for the needs of her family. When my father started having increased difficulty at work, his boss had to let him go. With my dad no longer employed, Mom had to begin working a night shift as a janitor cleaning high-rise buildings in downtown Los Angeles, as she tried to make ends meet. She worked through the night and then was home in time to get my brother and sister ready to meet their school buses by 6:30 am.

She was a hard worker and tirelessly pursued learning all she could about Huntington's Disease at a time when little was known about it. She attended conferences and in-services and met with numerous pediatricians, neurologists, and other specialists, searching for ways to make life more comfortable for my sister, brother, and Dad. In addition, Mom became a self-taught pharmacist as she studied the side effects of the myriad of medications that her family members would be prescribed over the next many years, learning which ones had an adverse impact on the disease.

When the care that my family members required was too much for Mom and me, she could no longer work. As a result, we became reliant upon various government assistance programs, friends, family, and our church community. Mom spent countless hours pursuing financial, medical, and respite assistance so she would not overly burden me as her assistant caregiver.

These journal entries from Mom sum up the overwhelmingly emotional experience that accompanied providing full-time care all those years.

*March 6, 1990*

*It was a week yesterday since Ron's death. It still seems impossible to even think of the world without him. The pain is so searing, so intense. It has no beginning, no end at this point—it does recede as unpredictably and erratically as it rushes over me, but seems only to recede—not go away. I miss him so terribly; I miss his smile, his voice, and being able to touch him, stroke his hair. My arms ache for that baby that lay in my arms, [who] learned to take first steps, say first words, ride a bike, use a wheelchair, accept being pushed in a chair, learned to use the toilet and learned to give up using the toilet—to open his mouth for food as a baby and be reduced to opening his mouth to be fed again as a young adult—but still smile—I find myself talking to myself—not out loud, but in my head. I tell myself—go thru the motions—it will get better; don't isolate yourself from life, from those who knew Ron—[because] thru them and thru me—he lives. I miss Ron, I miss Chrysty, and I miss Jerry; even though he hasn't left this life, he has left my life. I don't like the pain—it makes me so angry, and it hurts so much!*

*May 1990*

*I'm finding my feelings of loss of Chrysty are stronger again, as well…All I can see when I see their Dad is the gravestone and 3-tiered grave waiting for its final name and person. It is so very painful and I feel such loss—[with] my 2 children and my husband, who long ago became, in a strange way, another 'child' to me and the loss of their parts of the lives they might have had, and of the horrible pain each of them did live through—which Gerald still endures. It can be so overwhelming…*

*September 25, 1990*

*I seem torn where Lyndy's concerned. I feel I'm going through much of this torture and decision-making alone—not so much that someone else, Lyndy or anyone—could do it for me, but at least someone else would know what's happening.... She was there to at least some extent before—from a personal perspective on my part. The maternal part of me says—spare her and at the same time worries what she may have to endure (judging from past patterns) in the way of guilt for not having gone to see her Dad more often.*

*(From the journal of Judith Bohlin)*

A burden was lifted from me after reading her heartfelt entries. My mom, who I had looked up to and admired as a beacon of strength and hope all those years, had struggled. All those feelings and emotions of guilt, fear, anger, frustration, love, bitterness, and sadness that I had experienced over the years were not so unexpected after all and, indeed, had been something she was experiencing. Yet, her life was a testimony to the strength and resilience that God placed within her. She sought to help her affected family members and many others whose lives were touched by Huntington's Disease.

Mom fought for years to gain much-needed attention for HD so that funding and research could continue. She taught herself the nuances associated with the care given to those with Huntington's. She led in-services and forums and spoke at numerous events seeking to bring HD to the forefront of minds. In addition, she devoted much of her life to caring for the three affected family members within her own family, often sacrificing her health. With Dad's death, my mother sought to make the best of the person she had become. She remarried in 1999 to a dear friend, John (who also had extended family members with HD). Not only was he a close friend to our family, but he was like a father to my brother and me during the years our dad was in the state hospital. His support throughout those years was greatly needed and appreciated. Together, they served in various capacities with the Los Angeles Chapter of the Huntington's Disease Society of America. They led support groups, organized a large golf tournament fundraiser, and operated a hotline. So, when my mother's health began to decline, it was even more difficult to accept after seeing all of the sacrifices she had made, in caring for and advocating on behalf of those with HD.

Mom had a few brief "normal" years with her new husband, John, and time to spend with her new grandsons outside of a life focused solely on HD, but those years were still not easy. She struggled with her health while caring for John, and my grandfather, Poppo, both of whom had various health issues. In addition, the past years of physical care she gave had taken their toll— mentally and physically, as evidenced in some of her journal entries.

*November 1990*

*Now it's no longer clear that I'm not in the same place most people in our society are by my age, because of anything other than by my lack of getting myself there. My children are not here because of a disease process, not because I didn't do enough…But now that they're no longer here, it's difficult to make the connection. It simply feels as though I have arrived at this point in life with little to show for the years, for the work. I guess I need to do some things that will help to redefine my life, myself, both to me and to others, in that order. [In essence, she had to learn to make choices and decisions that were no longer based on the needs of others.] While I don't have complete choice, I surely have a lot more than ever before. So I guess it feels good, stranger, all kinds of things, at once. It also makes me feel incredibly sad—because it points to the fact, [and] brings [to] the surface the realization, that the reason this change has come about is that my children (along with their needs) are no longer here and that Jerry is living a miserable life away from his home. I know his life would be miserable at this point, in any case, but it is additionally so because he can't live in his home. I don't think I feel guilt about that—just sad and angry—at the loss of them all and to them all and to me. ... The change in circumstance gives me this freedom of choice; my freedom of choice is not responsible for my children's deaths—I remind myself, consciously of that whenever the feelings bubble up. They are not gone because of my increase in time to myself—the increase in time is here, because the conditions have changed.*

As mentioned earlier, I struggled with the guilt associated with not having HD. I now know my mom did as well. It affected her more deeply as a wife and mother on many different levels. She was able to move on with her life and find joy, but the skeletons and scars from the presence of HD in our lives remained.

*January 3, 1991* ———

*I remember saying to Lyndy at Disneyland on New Year's Day that I was just really discovering who I am without or outside the other role into which I've been cast in past/present—and that she may or may not like the person who is there—she may get to know me now instead of [me in] my role [as a caregiver]. I don't expect this me to be good or bad—just, maybe different—more multi-dimensional. I don't know how many people in my life, Lyndy included, will like dealing with and knowing me outside my usual more one-dimensional role in which they have related to me in the past. The discomfort, if there is any, will be their own difficulty in accepting/dealing with all of me—not my discomfort nor my changes.*

*March 13, 1991* ———

*I still feel so 'scattered.' I have a hard time concentrating, remembering names and things. Hardly a day on my calendar is left unscheduled, but when asked what I'm doing, I find it hard to give an answer—even to myself.*

———*(From the journal of Judith Bohlin)*

Mom continued to rebuild her life outside of HD by pursuing other interests she had been unable to consider previously. She began working as a chiropractic assistant and took some college classes, studying geology. She loved spending time with the boys and me, accompanying us on many homeschool field trips, and subbing as their teacher when I was sick. She and John designed and supervised rebuilding the house I grew up in (due to damage it had sustained from two separate earthquakes over the years). They attended concerts and plays and even went on vacations together. These were all things that she had put on hold for the past twenty-five years of her life. It was as if her life was now truly "normal."

CHAPTER TWELVE

# Here We Go Again

The normalcy in Mom's life was short-lived. Her health and that of my stepdad began to deteriorate. It wasn't until she had neck surgery in 2010 that we saw changes in her personality and overall demeanor. Suddenly, I noticed that she was ultra-focused on all things medical regarding herself or John. My mother's copious notes regarding the myriad of medications they took, as well as medical procedures and diagnoses, suggested a need to return to the life of being a caregiver. In addition, she herself began to show signs of possible hypochondriacism.

It seemed like she readily adopted the illnesses of those around her or even someone on television. But, whatever they had, she had it ten times worse. She started complaining of vomiting (in actuality, it was salivary reflux), began carrying a small bedpan with her wherever she went in case she needed to "throw up," and often refused to go out because of it. She also started to demonstrate other odd behaviors. Even though she had some issues with her balance, she refused to use a walker or cane because it "hurt" her fingers. She stopped using their new master bath because the grip bars near the toilet were "for handicapped people." Instead, she opted to use the guest bathroom down the hall. Later that year, over a three-day period, I received phone calls from all four of Mom's siblings expressing concern about her behavior and personality changes. Once extremely social, she now refused to speak with them on the phone.

She told people that her husband didn't want visitors when in reality, it was she who did not want them. Her sleep patterns changed. She stayed up all night, claiming she had to do so because of the medications she was taking, and then stayed in bed during the day until the afternoon. She began to lose the capability to recognize what was appropriate when it came to conversations (i.e., she would discuss her "vomiting" or bowel habits with people at dinner). At first, she only had these conversations with her immediate family. Still, they soon became commonplace as she would converse with anyone who made the mistake of asking, "How are you?" We later found that she had also been struggling to remember people she had known for years at the HD support groups and had become disinterested in attending them.

Instead of her usual pleasant stance, she began making a "wild-eyed" expression when posing for photographs. She referenced her physical ailments as "severe" and purchased different television remedies for memory enhancement. We later understood that these were symptoms associated with Frontotemporal Dementia (FTD). Other behaviors which were new for my mom, but typical for those with FTD, included hoarding and stockpiling. My parents' home became so overrun with trash that several rooms had only a path leading to the desk or bed. The countertops, ledges, bookcases, and any open surface, were covered with mounds of paper, odds and ends, pictures stacked on top of one another, and dust. In addition to a large quantity of "As Seen on TV" items, she kept both recent and expired Publisher's Clearing House mailings and copies of entries. Stacks of old Avon catalogs and unopened purchases in their bags sat on the treadmill. Reader's Digests, several decades of old paperwork stacked in boxes to the ceiling, and hundreds of empty plastic sacks, packages, and dry-cleaner hangers littered their home. When we attempted to assist with cleaning, she would comment, "Not today; I don't feel like it. Maybe when I feel better, I will get around to it." But that day never came. If I attempted to go and help clean some of the items from her closet, she would scream at me saying, "You are trying to kill me!" Eventually, John asked us to intervene. For three weeks, while they were out of town, my family, friends, and hired help stepped in to assist us in removing all the trash and accumulated items. During this clean-up, we located over 150 medications, some of which were not hers or expired, stockpiled, and even hidden throughout the house and garage.

I decided to speak with her doctor about the medications and supplements that she was taking which had been purchased from television ads. I hoped that perhaps he would agree to try to decrease the number of drugs so we could see if they were part of why her behavior and overall demeanor had changed. While he couldn't discuss her medical information with me at the time because she had not permitted him to do so, he was willing to at least listen to our concerns. In addition, after hearing what we were seeing, he could make better sense of what he had seen during many of the visits to his office. In the meantime, I convinced Mom (after much cajoling) to sign the necessary waiver, which would allow her doctor to speak with me. I provided a detailed list of all the medications found during the clean-up and spoke with him about the family's concerns regarding her recent behavior. As a result, the doctor agreed to discontinue some of her prescriptions and adjusted others. Unfortunately, Mom did not follow the doctor's orders and continued taking some of the old medications, thus making it difficult to tell whether they were indeed causing a problem.

The following year, in 2011, her primary physician referred her to a neurologist. During the initial examination, there were instances when Mom could not even answer simple questions. For example, the doctor asked her what holiday was coming up (Thanksgiving), but all she could answer was that it was a day that we ate a lot. When the doctor pointed to the watch she was wearing and asked her what it was, she replied, "I don't know, but it tells time." Later that day, she was diagnosed as having Frontotemporal Dementia. The doctor also noted that the medications she was taking could be exacerbating some of her current issues.

In retrospect, we could see that the subsequent changes in her personality and memory had begun sometime in 2007. According to the Mayo Clinic website:

Frontotemporal dementia is an umbrella term for a group of brain disorders that primarily affect the frontal and temporal lobes of the brain. These areas of the brain are generally associated with personality, behavior and language.

In frontotemporal dementia, portions of these lobes shrink (atrophy). Signs and symptoms vary, depending on which part of the brain is affected. Some people with frontotemporal dementia have dramatic changes in their personalities and become socially inappropriate, impulsive or emotionally indifferent, while others lose the ability to use language properly.

The most common signs of frontotemporal dementia involve extreme changes in behavior and personality. These include:

- Increasingly inappropriate social behavior
- Loss of empathy and other interpersonal skills
- Lack of judgment
- Loss of inhibition
- Lack of interest (apathy), which can be mistaken for depression
- Repetitive compulsive behavior, such as tapping, clapping or smacking lips
- A decline in personal hygiene

- Changes in eating habits, usually overeating or developing a preference for sweets and carbohydrates
- Eating inedible objects
- Compulsively wanting to put things in the mouth[6]

---

With the diagnosis of FTD, things started to make sense regarding her behavior. She had begun to demonstrate a severe paranoia of electricity, claiming it worsened her peripheral neuropathy. We spoke with the neurologist, who assured her there was no correlation. She continued to insist that it did cause a problem, but her reasoning made no sense. She avoided talking on the phone, walked a circuitous route around the Christmas tree, and wouldn't sleep on their adjustable bed because of electricity. She even insisted that a battery-operated card-shuffler be moved as far away from her as possible. Yet, she continued to use a curling iron, touch light switches, watch, and sit near the television even though these, too, had electricity.

By 2012, Mom's behavior and overall health worsened. Later that year, her father passed away. Even though she continued exhibiting changes in personality and memory, she was still capable of talking, carrying on a conversation, and writing. However, she did not display any emotion upon his passing other than simply acknowledging that he was gone as if she were a naïve young child. A few years prior, she had been a devoted daughter who had taken him to appointments and cared for him. Yet now, she wandered around the funeral home, busying herself in inappropriate ways.

I will never forget something that happened that night during the viewing. I was busy handling some of the details, which Mom would have previously done, when one of my aunts approached me and asked if I knew of Mom's recent actions. Unbeknownst to me, she had been making trips to the water cooler near the restrooms and was serving people cups of water. While this may not seem odd, she was, unfortunately, taking the paper cups from the trash can. When I tried stopping her, Mom said she had washed them out first. As I watched her change into a different person, I think this was when I started to acknowledge that, like my sister, brother, and father, she would not get better. As a result, my role in her care and the emotional turmoil of dealing with Mom's situation significantly increased.

*February 26, 2012*

*I have been attempting to go to Mom and John's for visits 2-3 times a week for the past month… we tried a caregiver service, but it was too expensive for someone who couldn't even help get her in the shower. It's frustrating not knowing what kind of activities mom might enjoy, as she shows little positive emotion. She seemed to enjoy the visit to Descanso [Gardens] and commented on different flower colors; but also became fidgety after about an hour and complained about walking. The aquarium was not as popular with her. I think it may have been due to the crowds intimidating her. John seems to really enjoy the outings—so despite her lack of excitement I am still determined to get her [and him] out [of the house.]*

*It's weird because I wonder if I am doing activities and such because it makes me feel better to think I am doing something; yet I do like to think that it is actually benefiting her because it is keeping her active and preventing her from drawing more and more into her shell and little world inside dementia.*

*Sometimes, though, I just feel like throwing my hands up and saying, "Fine, have it your way…stay in bed all day/night long!" but she didn't give up on raising me when I was difficult, and she didn't give up on continuously caring for her family members afflicted with HD even when symptoms were severe. So, I won't give up on her.*

*Even if she can't remember from one moment to the next what she did… I will remember for her.*

*Showering has become an issue…John struggles with getting her in—even once a week. He says he starts on Monday trying…and by Friday or Saturday, if lucky, he will finally get her in. It seems to help sometimes if we use what I call the good cop/bad cop [routine]…where John is the good one and I'm the bad one! We basically tell her Lyndy will come the next day and give her a shower if she doesn't get in with him.*

*July 29, 2012*

*Latest update with Mom: she was diagnosed a few months ago as being diabetic…I am guessing that in March, during what I am now calling "hell week," she had a bad problem with her blood sugar levels perhaps due to a UTI…this caused her to stay in bed all day and night and she refused to get up out of bed except to go to bathroom. She was also severely impacted [we later found out]. John was hospitalized that week with low oxygen levels…his body systems had started shutting down. [My husband and son had just had surgery but still had to stay with Mom while I was with John at the hospital.] The next day I tried to get her to come to our house and go to the doctor, but she refused. I could not get her to the car by myself. [So] I had to stay overnight with her. We needed to make sure she was taking the new diabetes meds [which she at first was not taking] and also the medicine for the infection.*

*Later entry* ———

*After being on Metformin [the new diabetes medication] for several months, we have seen an improvement and a return to "normal" for Mom. Normal being—at least getting out of bed. The only regular things we can get her to eat are peanut butter and jelly, some salad, fruit, applesauce, and chewy granola bars. She is still convinced that eating meat caused her to be impacted a few months ago, so since then, she has refused to eat meat. I can occasionally get her to eat some chicken if I put it in front of her, but if you ask her if she would like it in advance, she will say no.*

*It's funny when it comes to eating. I've learned that you cannot ask if she wants to eat something because she will usually tell you "no." After a lot of reading and attending some workshops, I have figured out that her response could be a result of her inability to make decisions anymore. So, if she just says "no," then she is still engaging in the conversation and showing some degree of power to act on her behalf. But, in reality, she does want the food. I have learned just to fix her small portions of what we are eating—IN ADVANCE—on her plate and then call her to the table. She will balk a little at first, then licks the plate clean! She will also quickly devour "undesirable" items, usually saving the regulars like peanut butter and jelly or salad till last.*

*We've seen a regression back to getting up later in the day, usually around 1 p.m. Unless we concentrate on getting her up and out and about, she will not do so on her own. John says that she is still wandering around at night [and even going outside by herself.] He often lays awake worried about what she is doing.*

*Several months ago, I convinced John to lock up all their drugs. After our last visit, the neurologist said it was no longer safe for Mom to take her meds without supervision. We can ensure what and how much she is taking by administering the medications. Unfortunately, John remains hesitant to totally take away her rights in this; so he still leaves Tylenol and her cups of meds out each day. I disagree. I think any medications she requires need to be given to her, period.*

*Regarding housing: we are still pondering what to do. It is apparent that John cannot totally care for mom … showering is an issue. She will only take one about every week and a half. She thinks she has just taken one...when in fact, it's been days. He is also unable to get her out for walks and is generally physically and emotionally tired. I think that dialysis is on the near horizon for him, and that will signal a change. At this point, we are hoping to find some inexpensive home care personnel to assist 3 times a week perhaps while he is at dialysis. This person can hopefully shower her, get her out for walks, make light meals for her, and be a companion/sitter while he is at dialysis.*

*All of this is taking an emotional toll on me. I feel as though I am needed by both of them, and am willing to help, as is Rob. However, we still have our own family and own health to be concerned with, so [we] are trying to figure out the best options for all involved. Unfortunately, those options are usually something that John and Mom don't agree with; or may not be able to afford. We had started the Medi-Cal process, but John hasn't been able to tie up all the loose ends for paperwork, so we still haven't succeeded in applying.*

*I feel like they look to me for help/answers...and I pray and try my best... but then sometimes my suggestions don't help or pan out. John assures me that it's not my burden to carry, and that they willingly made the decisions [regarding the different things we have tried] and were in agreement...so not to worry. What's done*

> *is done. But it's still hard, especially when it involves money that could have been used for care later. We spent it trying to get care, but when needed, we may not have it.*
>
> ——*From my journal*

I believe that it was during this "hell week" that my faith took a turn, as I became wholly dependent on God's strength. Later, I would see the many blessings that surrounded me despite the turmoil of emotional and physical exhaustion I experienced. I learned that not only did I need to turn to God, as I had already been doing in prayer, but I needed to trust Him to provide the strength I so desperately required. That trust meant I needed to actively look for and see what He was doing in my life and that of my parents. As a result, I became acutely aware of my need for His love manifested in many ways—often different from what I thought I needed or anticipated.

CHAPTER THIRTEEN

# I Just...Can't.

As we entered a new year, my mother's conduct markedly declined. Yet, years later, I would come to treasure her "behaviors" because they were reminiscent of a woman who could still talk, walk, and interact with the world around her: something that would later become nonexistent.

The year 2013 not only brought a deterioration in Mom's behavior, but our family also experienced a life-altering change. In June, I finished the arduous seventeen-year task of home-schooling the last of our three sons. After several weeks of my semi-retired state (I still worked at our summertime swimming business), I decided to investigate the possibility of returning to substitute teaching. That evening, as I sat on my computer checking out the details and preparing to submit my application, I received a phone call from John. He was lying in the street near their home, having fallen during an afternoon walk with my mom. He had called 911, and emergency personnel had arrived, but he didn't know what to do about her. She was not cooperating with them, and he was reasonably sure that the injury was severe enough to require being transported to the hospital. I immediately phoned the caregiver to see if she was available to tend to my mother while I headed to the hospital to meet the ambulance.

At this point, I had been more involved in both of my parent's medical care. I attended appointments, was the primary contact for their Advanced Healthcare Directive, and acted as their liaison with medical staff. Once I arrived at the hospital that day, I found that John had indeed severely broken his hip and was going to require surgery. I remember sitting there in the emergency room, trying to hold it together in front of him, as I started the task of apprising his four out-of-state children as to what had occurred and their father's current condition. My phone battery was dying, and I was struggling emotionally. I know I was uttering constant conscious and even unconscious prayers to God for strength and help. My mind was trying to grasp the magnitude of the situation, which looked pretty bleak.

Just about the time that I was ready to throw my hands in the air and crawl into a corner, pretending that none of this was happening, God heard me (well, actually, I know He heard my pleas for help all along, but this was a tangible sign I could cling to at the moment). He gave me the idea to reach out to my nearby sister-in-law to see if she had a phone charger I could borrow. She immediately came over and also brought me some food. As I sat in the waiting room, quietly crying, God had sent her as a beacon of hope. Finally, with some food in my stomach, a solid shoulder to cry on, and a now-charging phone, I could return to the situation at hand.

The doctors later determined that, while my stepdad did require hip replacement surgery, they would not be able to operate immediately due to his other medical conditions. He needed to be transferred to a different hospital and evaluated regarding the next steps. During the many hours that these various decisions took place, I determined that Mom would need to be relocated to our house, as the nurse could not stay with her full-time at my parent's home. The caregiver packed a suitcase for her, and my husband prepared for her arrival. Meanwhile, I continued to deal with the situation at the hospital. Upon being transferred, the new staff of doctors decided that the best option to prepare his body for surgery was to put him on a ventilator. The plan was to stabilize him and operate as soon as possible. He would then stay for recovery and subsequently enter a rehabilitation facility. This process would involve more than just a few nights away from home for him or Mom.

It would be an understatement to say that this event changed our lives. During what I thought was going to be a period in my life for me to start pursuing "life after surviving seventeen years of home-schooling," I felt like I was just trying to survive. When Mom arrived at our home, one of our sons graciously gave up his bed and slept on the couch for a few nights. I had spent several nights coming home emotionally and physically drained from long days at the hospital, crying out to God, wondering how on earth I was going from being newly "retired" to a life of, once again, becoming a caregiver. It was like a nightmare, deja-vu, except this time, it wasn't my mom who was the primary caregiver—it was me. As it became apparent that Mom would likely never be able to return to her home, Rob and I sat down to discuss our limited options. We prayed and felt that it was God's leading that we keep her at our house. However, we also laid out some guidelines. If caring for Mom became too physically challenging or potentially dangerous for me (or for her); caused problems in our marriage or immediate family; or if she became physically violent or required help beyond what we could give, we would pursue placement. We then sat down with our sons to explain our decision and ensure they were on board, and for the time being, her husband agreed with the plan.

Our three sons all lived at home at the time, so we had to make some quick renovations to our house to accommodate my mom. One son relocated to a different room since we decided that his bedroom would become hers. As hard as all the adjustments were for our family, I know they were even more difficult for Mom. I remember that for some time, I would go in to greet her in the morning and find her suitcase repacked. When asked why her bag was packed, she said she was going home. I would explain that this was her "home" now, but she didn't understand. It soon became a family affair as we each took "shifts" and learned how to care for Mom (Grandma). She tried to leave several times, so we had to put new locks on the front door that she could not access and on our backdoor so that she would not go out by the pool unassisted. Meanwhile, I continued to assist at the hospital with the various communication and advocacy needed on my stepdad's behalf. He eventually had his surgery, and the long process of recovery and rehabilitation began.

After the hospital, John was transferred to a skilled nursing facility and, eventually, an assisted living home. The next difficult hurdle we faced was the realization that neither he nor Mom would be able to return to their previous life or home. His physical limitations were such that he would be hard-pressed to care for himself, much less my mom. After conversations with his children, all of whom lived out of state, we decided to approach him with the suggestion that they both needed to consider placement or reside with us if they were to remain together.

To say that I felt strong in the Lord with all of the radical changes which occurred over a few months would be an overstatement. I felt lost. I wallowed in my "woe is me" moments quite frequently. I (nicely) railed against God, questioning His path for me. I couldn't fathom why I had to go through all this again. Didn't I give enough of my life to caregiving? I was desperate to find support, so I read various Christian books about caring for a sick parent. Many of these books talked about what a blessing it was to care for an aging or ill parent. I, however, just wasn't seeing that blessing on most days. His strength, I had only recently discovered, was now just a distant memory.

CHAPTER FOURTEEN

# The Emotional Roller Coaster

*And my God will meet all your needs according to the riches of his glory in Christ Jesus.* Philippians 4:19

Dementia is a devastating disease for the whole family. This excerpt from a speech my mother gave at a California Senate health committee hearing on June 16, 1995, regarding the dementia aspect of HD, says it well:

*I would like to try to 'personalize' the term 'dementia disorder' a bit for you. A dementia disorder, Huntington's Disease, in particular, has played a major role in shaping my life and the lives of my family members. My husband and two of our three children were afflicted with Huntington's Disease. Our two children are now deceased. Not many are familiar with Huntington's*

*Disease; even fewer are aware that the disease attacks young adults and children, as well as those in midlife.*

*Our daughter, Chrysty, first exhibited disease symptoms at age three and succumbed to Huntington's Disease just prior to her sixteenth birthday. Our son Ron's symptoms began appearing at about five to six years of age. He died an agonizing death at age 21. My husband, Gerald, has been symptomatic in excess of 20 years—much of our married life. Each of them was very 'normal' in every way prior to the onset of symptoms, which once underway, progress relentlessly to eventual death. I should underscore eventual death. In fact, it is very important to note that the progression of the disease—of most dementia diseases—is neither quick nor kind. Additionally, with HD, their person remains oriented and aware of the losses as they occur.*

As I watched my mother, who had once been a woman of such great strength, reduced to an adult who required the same care as a toddler, I battled an array of emotions.

- I struggled with not wanting to be too detached on an emotional level as a way of protecting myself, yet still wanting to be compassionate.

- I often felt defeated, frustrated, and even angry due to the lack of cooperation, as evidenced by my parents, as we tried to help.
- I felt the overwhelming pressure of wanting to be aware of our sons' needs as well as those associated with my marriage and personal health. I was determined not to let my caregiving duties affect my well-being to the extent they once had affected my mother.
- I wanted to be in God's will for my life, yet I struggled with feeling "stuck" in the situation.

*August 14, 2014*

*I don't know if it is Your will or mine that is making decisions. I feel as though what we are doing [caregiving] is right, but it also feels like there is more I could be doing [elsewhere] to use the skills You gave me. It's hard because it's as though I want to help others but sometimes don't feel like helping as much here at home, and I don't know if that's because it's too hard emotionally and physically or just because it's not my choice.*

—*From my journal*

I wondered at God's chosen answers to our prayers as we had been praying for a situation that would enable us to assist my parents (such as relocating nearer to us). But, that answer came in a way we hadn't anticipated with Mom's relocation to our home.

As mentioned previously, I struggled to find the "blessings" that so many others alluded to in the various books I read. For example, caring for my diabetic mother, who had several behavioral issues associated with dementia, and dealing with the emotional strain of the daily care related to these diseases was far from a "blessing" in my book.

A friend gave me an excellent book entitled "Just Enough Light for the Step I'm On" by Stormie Omartian. As I began to read, I was reminded that God is always at work in my life. He wants me to call out His name and ask Him to direct me. As I refocused my eyes, spiritually and literally, I started seeing my position differently. I noticed the blessings amidst the hardships, anger, sorrow, and distress. Finally, I was able to start finding joy in my situation.

I found that in the Bible, joy and sorrow are often linked together.

*Very truly I tell you, you will weep and mourn while the world rejoices. You will grieve, but your grief will turn to joy.* *John 16:20*

*We can rejoice, too, when we run into problems and trials, for we know that they help us develop endurance. And endurance develops strength of character, and character strengthens our confident hope of salvation. And this hope will not lead to disappointment. For we know how dearly God loves us, because he has given us the Holy Spirit to fill our hearts with his love."*

*Romans 5:3-5 (New Living Translation)*

I found this same "joy linked to sorrow" in my caregiving journey, and as a result, I eventually did see His blessings.

*October 24, 2014* ———

*I think I find joy linked to sorrow in my caregiving when I see the changes in mom. It's hard to see her now, knowing she was a vibrant, caring, go-getter. But I have learned to look for new things in this season of her life that bring her joy, like seeing Shamu, playing cards, and listening to music. I have also experienced joy as I watched the boys and Rob care for her. I am saddened by the fact that we must go through this, but also joyful knowing it has matured them and brought us closer together as a family.*

——————————————————*From my journal*

I experienced joy in many ways:

- Watching our sons contribute to my mother's care. They each took turns "grandma-sitting" so Rob and I could have date nights and weekends away. They sacrificed their time, gave up their bedrooms, and moved into a hastily-built shed in our backyard. Knowing that they "had my back" also brought joy to me as I saw Christ at work in them. Despite the sadness associated with seeing their grandma's deterioration, they were still maturing and becoming godly young men who demonstrated compassion as they helped care for her.
- Learning to write down positive aspects of our situation instead of focusing only on the negative. I began to see that, all along, God's hand had indeed been gently resting on me. He had been providing for, and more importantly, blessing, us. I saw that Rob and I had grown closer to one another, both as husband and wife and as best friends and helpmates. We weathered the storm together, thus

strengthening our marriage more than I imagined or could have desired.

- Gaining new friends the Lord faithfully brought across my path, each of whom had a parent with dementia.
- Seeing that not only was I being obedient to God's call on my life, but I was also providing help and care for my mother, as she had done for me in so many ways over the years.

As time progressed, I learned to create new "memories," which would later help combat the times of frustration and sadness surrounding our situation. One of my fondest recollections after Mom was diagnosed with dementia was when we took her to Sea World. My husband and I planned a trip to take her and John for an overnight visit to San Diego. We were able to take a caregiver along who would assist them during the overnight portion and help during the day while at the park. Until then, my mom had stopped displaying any emotion except anger over things we did to try to help her. One of the highlights of the day was the Shamu show. During the pre-show, she became very animated as the music began to play. She started clapping and tried to get the rest of us to join. When the show started, she became enthralled by the jumping and splashing of the killer whales. She not only exclaimed her enjoyment, but she showed it. She smiled and laughed, which was something she had not done for several years. She loved it. In fact, throughout the rest of the day, she even asked to return to the show! When we went to the underwater viewing area to see the whales, she stood in awe as she touched the glass to "talk" to them. It was indeed a happy moment for her and the rest of us. Now, instead of allowing the challenging moments to overshadow the more joyful memories as I had often done, I chose to remember treasured moments like this. I would cling to the combination of newly created memories and answered prayers as the roller coaster ride known as dementia continued.

Even though some of these blessings were in disguise at the time, they were blessings, nonetheless. God was and would continue to be there, demonstrating His mercies every day. I just had to stop and take the time to see them. I knew God was with me all along, but as I like to say, "It's so easy to wallow instead of follow!" It wasn't until I took the emphasis off of me and began to focus on the blessings that He bestowed upon me that I was able to drag myself up out of the pit of despair and proceed with praising and thanking God instead. My situation didn't change, but I did. My walk with Him grew stronger as I faced each day. Not only did I have a keen sense of my need for God's presence in my life, but I also recognized that He was constantly providing for me and that He loved me. As I realized His many blessings, my praise to and for Him became sweeter.

*August 2014*

*Lord, I am reminded by your word that—*

*I will give you hidden treasures, riches stored in secret places, so that you may know that I am the LORD… who summons you by name.* Isaiah 45:3 (NIV)

*I know that during this time of caring for my parents, you are giving me "hidden treasures" and drawing me closer. I know You are helping me to grow closer to You and to grow in my faith. Help me to see the blessings You provide instead of continuously fretting about what the future holds and all the "what ifs." I know I worry about what we will do with Mom when the time comes to place her—help me just to trust that You will continue to guide us, as You have already done, and provide (like giving us caregivers we know and trust and even respite money to help!) Thank You.*

———————————————————*From my journal*

*August 14, 2014* ———————————————————

*[Lord] we are unsure about mom's care at this point and don't know if we should pursue looking for homes. Help us to know which direction to head. If she should stay here, then I ask that we be able to find some consistent care that can be here more often, if needed, especially because of the toileting and showering… [this prayer was answered almost immediately as we were able to find a great agency that provided the additional help we needed consistently, and at affordable rates] … If it is time to consider placement then I ask that You provide just the right home for her. One that will fit their budget, provide adequate supervision, great care, and activities to keep her engaged and easy enough for us to visit still. I know I look at this as a monumental, and at times unattainable, task when it comes to locating a good home—but I know You are bigger than all that and that Your light will give me all the help I need if I just trust You to help me. [This prayer was answered about a year later.]*

———————————————————*From my journal*

*"I remain confident of this: I will see the goodness of the LORD in the land of the living. Wait for the LORD; be strong and take heart and wait for the LORD."*

*Psalm 27:13–14*

CHAPTER FIFTEEN

# Riding the Roller Coaster

After several months of living with us, Mom had reluctantly begun to accept that our home was now her home. She stopped repacking her suitcase every day, and we started the task of creating routines that would hopefully help diminish some of her anxiety about her new life. We knew she was confused, especially regarding the absence of her husband; however, taking her to visit him in the hospital proved to be too difficult due to her behavior. Once he had his surgery and subsequently moved to a skilled nursing facility and an assisted living home, we could more readily take her to see him.

When we weren't visiting him or attending doctor's appointments, we created ways to include her in our daily lives. One of the first tasks we attempted was to set up a routine addressing Mom's physical hygiene, which had previously been an area of contention. For example, I created a chart that showed which days we would help her take a shower (in addition to other events during the day like appointments, activities, meals, and nap times). She often felt that she did not need to shower since, in her mind, she had just done so. Though Mom was still mobile at this point, she required some assistance with most daily routines, including showering, toileting, and dressing.

Our next goal was to get her diabetes under control. I monitored what she ate, and we took turns trying to increase her activity level. Part of our daily schedule included walks with her using her walker. When we first mentioned the idea, she said, "no." However, we insisted. Short walks in front of the house soon evolved into journeys throughout the neighborhood for long periods of time.

We spent time playing her favorite card game, "May I." I tried to involve her in exercise using the "Nintendo Wii" game system. She and I worked together doing basic word searches or painting pictures. Now, instead of staying in bed till the early afternoon, our goal was to help her follow a more suitable schedule which included waking at a set time in the morning, taking a nap, engaging in activities throughout the day, and heading to bed at a set time. She even attended church with us on Sundays and enjoyed listening to the worship music, though, at times, her behavior was inappropriate. We quickly determined that "life," although different, needed to go on for her and us.

As the months progressed, it was apparent that caring for Mom had become my full-time job. I remember days that I cried out to God, telling Him I just couldn't do it anymore. Attending to her was physically and emotionally draining, not to mention time-consuming. Yet, God again reminded me of His presence and provision during these moments.

The year before John's accident, I had the opportunity to reconnect with a young woman whom I had known since she was four. She and her sister were the same ages as our sons, and we all attended the same church. Over the years, we had lost touch, but God, in one of His "I've got you" moments orchestrated the crossing of our paths. As we chatted, I discovered she was pursuing becoming a nurse and wanted to focus on in-home care! I explained what was happening with "Grandma Judy" (as they had known her), and what followed is a treasured example of God's provision and timing. Within months, she became a caregiver to my mom (while they still lived in their home), assisting John a few days a week and accompanying them, on occasion, for outings. Once Mom resided with us, she continued to provide care at our home. She had completed her CNA training and worked for a hospice organization which later accepted my mother as a client. I cannot tell you what a huge blessing this was for our family and me. Not only had God provided someone we fully trusted with Mom's care, but a significant portion of her hours and an additional CNA were covered financially. God also provided friends who offered to come and sit with my mom and entertain her so I could do basic tasks like go to the grocery store. They were a godsend because it had become increasingly difficult to take her with me to the market due to her grabbing items and combative behavior.

After a few months, our lives settled into a new rhythm. Each day brought new challenges, but we were confident and met them head-on. However, this "rhythm" was soon interrupted by the news that John had completed his rehabilitation and was ready to come live with us. His impending arrival brought further changes to our home and lives.

We decided that since our home would now become their home, we needed to figure out a way for them to have a private living space. Until then, it had worked well just to use one bedroom for my mother because she accompanied us throughout the day. If we were in the living room, she sat there with us. If we were preparing meals, she was nearby at the table. However, my stepdad's presence now meant that he would, in theory, become her primary caregiver regarding supervision. Our only option was to renovate the adjacent bedroom so they could use one bedroom as their "living quarters" with comfortable recliners, end tables, television, desk, and wardrobe. The other bedroom became their sleeping quarters with two hospital beds, a temporary toilet, and a sink area my husband created from a closet.

Meanwhile, all three of our sons still resided at home, so we quickly developed an alternative living space for them to live. Our newly renovated master bathroom had a walk-in shower, so it was the only shower my parents could use. We had to add grab bars to make it safe for their use. I guiltily struggled emotionally with all these changes. Even something as basic as adding those grab bars to the shower was a HUGE thing. In my mind, I pictured a little "devil" version of myself sitting on one shoulder, saying, "It's so unfair that the aesthetics of my new beautiful bathroom are marred by shower chairs and grab rails." In contrast, the little "angel" version sat on the other shoulder, saying, "Think about all the changes your parents are going through! How petty and selfish can you be!" Essentially, part of me viewed it as another sacrifice, which became one more reason for me to whine about the unfairness of my situation to God.

I'm amazed at God's grace and patience when we act humanly. Once again, I was so focused on myself that I was not focusing on God. I trusted in and fell back on my strength and capabilities to get through the situation. I could fix this. I would be the savior my parents needed in their moment of need. Unfortunately, I wasn't looking to gain my strength from Him, nor was I fully trusting Him to provide for them and my family. A journal entry I wrote after the fact illustrates this attitude well.

*January 27, 2021*

*Just like [my grandson] smiling as he is pushing me out the door to the rec room so that he could either go in the garage [where he wasn't supposed to go] or use the [forbidden] remote—I am like that with You, God. I gently nudge You behind the door and close it while smiling at You as if I am just fine—so that I can attempt to do what I want to do, when I want to do it. But that almost always winds up placing me in situations where You did not want me. Help me to keep the door wide open with my eyes on you...trusting that You know what's best and [that] You will let me go on that walk [or in that room] when You are ready to take me there.*

—*From my journal*

Because of my myopic view, I couldn't see the forest for the trees. Each little hiccup in my "plan" to navigate daily life seemed like a mountain to climb; instead, it was simply a speed bump that I allowed to throw me off course. God wanted to guide and provide for me. I just wasn't listening as clearly as I should have been. As I realigned my thinking alongside His, I found a calming presence and stability. We could figure out living arrangements for our sons, and thanks to my fantastically-talented husband, we provided an excellent area for my parents to live in for almost two years. (Despite my selfishness, God even allowed me to have my beautiful bathroom back a few years later!)

Our lives now settled into yet another new routine. My parents hung out in their sitting room, watching television together in the afternoons. They seemed content for the most part. Subsequently, Rob and I had some time to ourselves and resumed leading a church group that had previously met at our home. During the morning, I assisted caregivers in showering Mom and taking her for walks. Occasionally, I would play cards with Mom and John. I still provided all their meals, and we usually ate together as a family. My parents even went out to dinner and a few plays accompanied by a caregiver. In some regards, my family was able to resume part of what I would say was our previous "normal" life: pre-parents-moving-in.

When we agreed to have my parents live with us, I expected that there would be challenges. I knew there would be adjustments and sacrifices because I knew what I had relinquished as a teenager/adult and had witnessed, first-hand, all my mother had given up to care for our family. Therefore, I felt as though I "rolled with the punches" as we learned to care for Mom after she moved in. However, I would soon discover a newfound need to rely even more extensively on God's strength as we now had both of my parents there with us—for reasons I couldn't have imagined.

CHAPTER SIXTEEN

# The Plummeting Drop

My stepdad loved my Mom. He was whole-heartedly devoted to her and made the tough choice to give up their home and move in with us so they could stay together. Unfortunately, despite this great love for her, he had difficulty providing the level of care she required.

Before moving in with us, he had already been struggling emotionally and physically to give the extensive assistance she needed. I think he found it very hard to accept that she had dementia and felt that everything would be okay if he just "ignored" its presence. For the most part, he and I had previously worked well together, but in retrospect, I think this was because we were on the same "team" when dealing with my mom's needs. I loved him as if he were my biological father and knew he loved my family and me. But, as Mom's dementia worsened, I had to take a more active role in her care. My increased involvement slowly started eating away at the cooperative spirit my stepdad and I had enjoyed. For example, while they were still living in their home, I devised a whole picture-coded system to assist John with preparing meals conducive to managing my mom's diabetes. Yet, he eventually gave in to her desires and allowed her to predominantly eat foods that were not good for her because it was just too much of a battle. When we attended her next nutritionist appointment, the dietician pointedly told me that I needed to get her eating under control or she would have to begin using insulin. I was disappointed that he wouldn't use the system I had devised. As a result, I continued to express my concern regarding my mom's eating habits.

I had other notable areas of concern before they moved into our home. I had expressed my fears regarding her (and his) safety. He had told me about an instance while preparing for Halloween trick-or-treaters. He tried to outline what would happen during the evening, explaining that some children would come to the door and knock, and she would help give them some candy. She nodded in agreement but then disappeared into the kitchen. A few moments later, she came out carrying two large knives and placed one by his chair and the second one by hers. She told him that this was in case they needed them to protect themselves. She didn't understand that the visitors coming to their door were innocent children. Following this occurrence, I suggested that he lock the drawers with the sharp knives in case she one day failed to remember who he was and subsequently tried to "protect" herself. Again, he said it was "fine" and did not see the need to do so.

After many months of ongoing discussions, my husband and I convinced my stepdad that they needed help if they were to continue living in their home. As part of that process, my husband and I ensured that legal necessities like powers of attorney, joint bank accounts, and an irrevocable trust were implemented. Next, we began the arduous process of applying for Medi-Cal (which could be a book in and of itself)! Our entire family had become part of a "team" that worked together to help my mom as her dementia progressed. However, all of that changed when they moved in with us. The dynamics quickly switched from a "team emphasis" to an "us against them" perspective as we started to see and feel the unhappiness that my stepdad was exhibiting.

With John's arrival at our home, we had started to notice that, though he tried to help keep an eye on my mom, it wasn't always enough. My mom's diabetes was under control, but she still needed constant monitoring regarding her ability to sneak into the kitchen for food and inedible things. Soon, the chain we had placed across the hallway proved inadequate as she learned to crawl under it and down the hall to the kitchen. In addition, the motion alarms we tried didn't always give us the time to respond quickly enough to stop her from getting into restricted areas. Eventually, we had to place an additional door in the hallway. My stepdad didn't like feeling like they were shut-in—even though we had always offered that they could come and join us for movies, etc., as long as there wasn't a group function in progress.

Unfortunately, my mom's behavior had worsened considerably and required much more attention than it had previously. She was becoming more combative in the kitchen during meals (trying to take food from other people's plates and the pantry). Eventually, we had to resort to serving their meals in the sitting room to protect against easy access to the refrigerator and cabinets. Her inappropriate behaviors in public became so problematic that taking her out had become too challenging. We could not take her to church anymore due to occasions where she pulled the hair of someone in front of us and tried to go up on stage during the service (becoming combative when we attempted to stop her).

Eventually, we had to employ the assistance of an agency for help on Sunday mornings since it was too tricky for my stepdad to monitor my mom at the level she required. The reality was that she and her husband could no longer go out even with a caregiver. I know that all of this, combined with the necessary limitations we had in place, weighed heavily on my stepdad. Despite my dear uncles' efforts to take him out occasionally for meals and drives, I know that the walls must have seemed as though they were closing in on him.

Since one of our primary stipulations at the beginning of this caregiving journey was to maintain a healthy marriage, Rob and I had decided to take a vacation now that we were not the sole primary caregivers for my mom. It involved considerable planning on our part regarding her care. We arranged caregivers, and if one of our sons was unavailable overnight, we had to ensure someone else could be there to assist my parents as needed. Upon our return, we found that my stepdad had dismissed or canceled some of the caregiving we arranged and felt he should no longer have to pay for it. His reaction, coupled with the fact that my mother's dementia was in a state of rapid decline, signaled that change was on the horizon. Notes from my care journal illustrate the advanced stage her dementia had reached.

*As of August 2013, there were still glimpses of the mom I had known all my life, but we began to see further deterioration and behaviors:*

- *She didn't know what clouds were (she said they were "white things in the sky")*
- *She tried to "cool off" her curling iron by running it under water (thankfully wasn't plugged in!)*
- *Still seemed to know grandsons, but not names*
- *Still knew I was her daughter*
- *Talked about her first husband and children (not by name) that died from something and how she was glad that I didn't get it*
- *Knows Rob and I, but not usually names*
- *Still calls John by his name*
- *Could still sign name*
- *Seemed to enjoy doing word searches; simple addition problems; watching Jeopardy and Wheel of Fortune (she would even mimic the announcer by saying, "Here's Vanna")*

*Even those abilities, however, didn't last for long. By 2014 she exhibited the following:*

- *John, her husband, is more often referred to as "her man" instead of by name*
- *Rob is "my [Lyndy's] man" (and not called Rob)*
- *Knows boys are my sons but no longer realized they were her grandsons*
- *She could still do word search puzzles and simple addition fairly well and still write her name*
- *She doesn't recognize herself in pictures*
- *Enjoys playing "May I" (obsessive at times and often changes rules to suit her)*
- *Wants food all the time. It became such a problem that we had to put up barriers to the kitchen (we progressed from a chain across the kitchen doorway to a chain with bells and eventually resorted to an audible motion alarm)*
- *Trying to eat non-edible items (fall candles, Christmas tree, small rubber balls, hand sanitizer) and paper, which led to vomiting*
- *Paces back and forth to get "it" to come down before going to the bathroom*
- *Has stuck a hand in the toilet to touch feces*

*By 2015 many skills, which had been present up until now, were almost non-existent:*

- *Began calling most things "trees"*
- *She doesn't know her name*
- *She still likes to count items, but not sure if she can do addition anymore*
- *Will try word search puzzles, but she is very "creative" at how she finds the words*
- *She still played "May I" but has increasing difficulty with the rules of the game and makes up her own rules as she goes along*

CHAPTER SEVENTEEN

# One of the Hardest Decisions Ever

*January 27, 2015*

*We are now entering the second year of having mom and John live with us. It has not been without its trials. Things came to a head a few weeks ago, and John said he was moving out and taking mom… or leaving her… wasn't sure. Said he wouldn't pay for caregivers anymore either.*

*—From my journal*

In the back of my mind, I think I always knew that we would eventually have to place my mom. It was the scenario I dreaded because I felt I would be failing her. So, the superhero in me continued to pray that God would somehow rectify the situation we now found ourselves in; or, conversely, show us a way out of it. But unfortunately, with my stepdad's increasing unhappiness came tension. Our relationship was strained, and though we had conversations and tried to figure out how to improve it, it was fruitless. I know he didn't blame us, but his sense of feeling caged was proving to be too much for him to bear.

After several years of dealing with the ever-changing dynamics of dementia and all it entails, I had learned to look for God to act. I had seen his provisions and was trusting Him daily. Instead of seeking to fix the situation in my strength (as I had so quickly done in the past), I was acquiring the capability to rely on His strength. We had prayed that He would somehow show us when and if it was time to place my mom should the need arise. In His faithfulness, He did just that.

*March 2015* ———

*Rob noticed her eating something...When removed from the mouth it appeared to be toilet paper. Of course, we were concerned—so Rob questioned John, and it was brought to our attention. that mom was [and had been, unbeknownst to us, for several weeks] eating toilet paper. Once our home nurse was told, she expressed concern over it and stated that it could cause bowel obstruction. She also noted that she would [need to] inform her administrator [with the hospice] and that we could be found liable if we weren't doing something to stop her [my mother]. Rob contacted our friend, who works in the social worker system, and she advised that we start looking for placement because mom required supervision beyond what we (and John) could provide. The hospice director also suggested the same, and her doctor concurred that it was a wise decision. We could now see that we would no longer be able to provide the necessary care for her.*

———————————————————*From my journal*

Finding a suitable home nearby that provided memory care, and accepted Medi-Cal, was grueling. My dear husband spent much time checking out facilities, but none seemed like what we wanted. It was depressing since many appeared dreary and impersonal. At this point, I would like to insert, once again, that God amazed me with His provisions. My extended family was well aware of the situation and supported our decision to place my mom. Soon after we began our search, Mom's brother and sister-in-law called me. They suggested I reach out to their brother-in-law, an administrator at a local assisted living facility with a relatively new memory care center! Of course, I quickly made the call, only to find out that we would have to place her on a waitlist and to expect that it could be many months before a "Medi-Cal" bed became open. Unfortunately, those were not the words we wanted to hear, but we maintained hope and continued to pray.

*June 25, 2015*

*We were impressed from the beginning with the facility. After having toured other homes, we knew that it was, by far, one of the nicest. The staff was caring, attentive, and knowledgeable. There were activities offered during the various times of day that we visited, and [we] loved the idea that mom would be able to wander and even walk freely outdoors in a secured garden area alone. This was something she had been unable to do safely at our home. In addition, we were confident that she would be closely monitored and that this staff was trained to handle her various behaviors.*

*Unfortunately, the road to making the placement a reality was not a smooth one.*

*With the circumstances that had occurred, it was clearly a sign from God that it was indeed time. The fact that my aunt and uncle had recommended that we call their brother-in-law; and the fact that the facility took Medi-Cal seemed like additional signs that it was indeed the right choice. Further cementing the decision… was another "God moment" when a caregiver from Right at Home [our current agency for at-home care] came to replace the previous one…and chatting with her, we found out that she worked at the memory care unit [at that same facility]! So now we knew an additional person who would know mom.*

*After touring the facility, we were convinced that it was the nicest place we could find for mom and had no qualms about placing her there. We felt it was indeed an answer to our prayers.*

———————————————*From my journal*

A favorite Bible verse I turned to throughout this process was:

*Have I not commanded you? Be strong and courageous. Do not be afraid; do not be discouraged, for the LORD your God will be with you wherever you go.*

*Joshua 1:9*

I truly felt that Rob and I had honored my parents and our Lord by following His Word and helping to care for them during the years we did. As we prepared to enter this next phase of assisting them, it was comforting to be reminded of His presence with my mother and us wherever we went.

Roughly three months after placing my mom on the waitlist, we received the go-ahead for an intake interview to see if Mom was a good candidate at this facility. Now that placement was a tangible reality, I remember crying out to God, and my husband, expressing my doubts over our impending decision. Thankfully, God gave me an angel-in-disguise in the form of the sweet head nurse who performed the intake. She helped me understand that because my mom could no longer speak for herself, I (we) had to be her advocate. We had to ensure that she was in a safe environment, ultimately enabling her to thrive. This particular memory care unit was "state-of-the-art" and designed to help those with dementia feel "at home." We felt God had given us the affirmation we needed in more ways than one.

*June 25, 2015*

*For months, we would check in every few weeks to see if there was any progress or how much she had moved up on the waitlist. In June, we received a heads-up that a spot may become available, but it was given to an internal candidate [this had also been something that had hindered her progress on the waitlist]. We got another* *call a few weeks later, but it did not happen again. We were warned that when it did happen, if it was not the end of the month, then a bed hold (costing a little over $300 a day) would have to be done until the end of the month, as insurance (which she would have to be disenrolled from) could not be transferred until [then]. We received the call on June 16 stating that a bed was finally available. We accepted the spot and began the process of trying to secure it. We had to pay for 17 days of holding the bed up front since it happened mid-month. We were then told that she was no longer showing that she was enrolled in Medi-Cal and that we would have to start that process again.*

*Several years previously, we had gone through a long process of applying for Medi-Cal using a hired agency that assisted us. They successfully got both of my parents into the Medi-Cal system, but their [my parents'] share of the cost was quite high [approximately 86% of their income]. However, over the few years between that process and the actual placement, something had happened that resulted in my mother no longer appearing in their system.*

*Rob spent hours on the phone (every time he called in, he had to go through numerous recordings, each requesting various information, which would* *eventually get you to a live person). After speaking with multiple individuals, we received several versions of their actual status in the Medi-Cal system. For example, one person told him my stepdad was living in long-term care [which he was not], and yet another said my mother already was! A third person said the share of the cost was "$200ish," while a different person said it was "$2400ish." Finally, after speaking with the rep at the Jewish home, he was told he better go ahead and start reapplying for Mom as she was not finding an active account.*

*Several long days were spent completing the same paperwork that had been done years prior, and we had it reviewed by a case worker at the Jewish Home. She then gave him more paperwork to fill out, which would assist in possibly getting some retroactive reimbursement for caregivers we had used in the home. (Something which we had repeatedly tried to get but had been told that their share of cost precluded them from receiving that kind of assistance!)*

*After thinking we were finally on the road to being ready for a July 1 move-in date, we found out that the doctor had not checked off a necessary box that would ensure that this was the correct placement for mom. Back in February, he had completed the very same form required to begin [the process of] placing her on the waiting list. But then, since the wait had taken beyond three months, that form had to be completed again. There was a misunderstanding regarding the wording, and after a few phone calls, he did sign and submit the form.*

*We also had to disenroll mom from her insurance. Again, Rob spent hours on the phone. The first person he spoke with told him to go online and fill out a form that could be immediately submitted online. When he attempted to do so, there was no such form. However, one was located that could be printed out and mailed in. After calling back and explaining his dilemma and the urgency of getting it completed (to a different person), she offered to submit it herself.*

*As we continue on this path, I am finding that it has been a time of growth and struggle in my faith. I sometimes question if we are doing the right thing because we felt led to do so, but then once we began, we have had nothing but problems. After continued prayer, though, I was reminded that I was never truly thankful for the fact that a bed became available! I have seen the necessity of focusing on the positive things to be grateful for, and trying to rest in the fact that, God has provided all along the way. Sometimes that provision has not been what we expected, or in the timing we had anticipated, but it was provided. I was reminded this morning of this verse:*

*...And we boast in the hope of the glory of God. Not only so, but we also glory in our sufferings, because we know that suffering produces perseverance; perseverance, character; and character, hope. And hope does not put us to shame, because God's love has been poured out into our hearts through the Holy Spirit, who has been given to us.*

*Romans 5:2-5*

*This process has been one of perseverance, especially on my dear husband's part. God has provided him as my "physical rock,"—someone to give me the help, love, and support I need most...in a tangible way. God has been my all-providing rock in hope, strength, and faith.*

———————————————*From my journal*

God answered so many prayers in those few months that I still marvel at how He moved on our (and my mother's) behalf. Even with the various speedbumps slowing down our progress, He smoothed our path by enabling Rob to reach the correct people at Medi-Cal, doctor's offices, and the Jewish Home who would help facilitate the placement. We even received another answer to prayer, which was massive praise in the form of a phone call a day after she was placed. They decided that since we had made the new application for Medi-Cal in June, they would honor it, return our check for $9,000+ for July's rent, and charge us only the estimated share of the cost ($500-600).

July 1, 2015 is a day that will forever remain etched in my mind. It was the day that we finally moved my mom to the facility. I would venture to say that it was one of the hardest things I have had to do (and I wasn't the one who had to take her there). We had already taken whatever items we could to prepare her room with familiar things that could help her acclimate to the new surroundings. Even this was not an easy task because we still had to keep her room at our home somewhat "normal" for her until it was time to move. The head nurse briefed us on the protocol and suggested how to facilitate the move. She explained that it was best for someone who could remain unemotional to bring mom because if she sensed something was wrong, she would become concerned. Upon her recommendation, we decided that my husband Rob would take her.

*July 3, 2015* ———

*Well, mom has been placed in the Jewish Home. Rob took her over on the morning of July 1. He said it was not an easy task. Emotionally, he was o.k., till [the administrator] came over and Rob said we would be going to the cabin.*

———————————————*From my journal*

That she would not be accompanying us on this trip, as she had previously done, was an unexpected emotional realization for Rob that hit home at that moment. My mother noticed him getting teary-eyed and subsequently became upset. For the remainder of the day, the staff said she kept trying to leave.

We did go ahead and go to our cabin that weekend because another part of the check-in routine at the facility stressed that it was best that the family not visit during the first few weeks after placement. This process more readily facilitated the resident's acceptance of the new location as their home. It was an extremely emotional time for us for many reasons. First, the fact that we had gone through with my mom's placement was finally becoming a reality. Second, I was heartbroken after hearing that my husband had struggled with taking my mom. Third, as we called to check in those first few days, it became increasingly harder to hear that she was stressed (as many residents are at first). She was trying to leave the facility, wandering around the unit, attempting to open all the doors, and was often combative. Each of these reports served as constant "needles" that pricked at me and my conscience. The "what if" questions resurfaced, and the Enemy tried to make me believe I was failing as a daughter. God, however, girded me and held me up as he surrounded me with my husband, sons, and extended family, all of whom supported my decision. His faithfulness was apparent throughout those years as I entered the next phase of caring for my mom.

CHAPTER EIGHTEEN

# The Long & Winding Road

Once we began visiting my mom in her new place, one of the first things she said to us was sad yet humorous. My son, husband, and I accompanied her on a walk around the beautiful grounds. As Mom greeted the various statues we passed (something she loved to do), she stopped, looked at us, and said she didn't know how she got there. Then she stated, in an indignant manner, that "Some guy brought me here, and then just left me!" In that rare moment, we were thankful for the memory loss that made it, so she didn't realize it was Rob! During those first few months, it was still a struggle for Mom: her behavior continued to express itself differently. She stole food from other residents, paced around the floor, and reverted to staying in bed during the day.

*July 2015*

*It's a little disheartening when we come and find her in bed. We worked so hard to keep her from spending all her time in bed, even though most of the time it was watching tv, walking, or playing May I. I am hopeful that she will become more cooperative with the staff's attempts to engage her in activities and that the staff will be a little more insistent.*

*July 14, 2015*

*Mom has calmed down at the Home. At first, she kept pacing and trying to find ways out. They said she would go to the payphone and [phone at the] nurse desk, push buttons, and then say, "It wasn't working." She asked to call John on the first day I went to visit. She wanted to know the name of the city the place was in so she could tell him how to get there.*

Over the next month, she seemed as though she was settling in, and we collectively felt relieved. However, it was short-lived.

*While we know it was the right thing to do for her and us; it was so hard. The most challenging part is hearing that she is scared and confused. We just continue to pray that God's peace that passes all understanding will surround her and that she will find staff who are sympathetic and caring, who take the time to try to figure out what will comfort her.*

*God brought to mind that her wishes (as stated in her Advanced Directive from 2010) were that measures be taken to help make her life comfortable and as good as it could be…that she wanted measures taken to allow her to live. That is what we have done by making this choice.*

—*From my journal*

As of September 2015, she no longer knew who we were by name, still seemed to enjoy visits from her family and taking walks around the campus, but no longer desired to play her favorite card game. Unfortunately, her behavior only worsened.

In October 2015, Mom was placed on a 72 hour psychiatric hold, which meant they had to call and have her removed from the unit and placed in a psychological ward due to her aggressive behavior exacerbated by her constant desire for food. Once again, we could not visit her while she remained on this unit as they sought to make medication adjustments to help alleviate some of the behavioral symptoms. As her primary caregiver/

representative, it was stressful because I had to approve using different medications. Given that I felt that the vast number of medications my mom had taken over the years had contributed to her current situation, this was not an easy decision. God provided help in the form of my sister-in-law, a pharmacist, who helped guide me through deciphering and understanding what symptoms each of the medications addressed. Added to that stress was the constant concern that, should she be gone too long from her new "home" we would have to start paying the total amount to hold her bed because Medi-Cal only allowed for her to be absent for a short pre-determined period. The cost of her current living space was almost $10,000 a month. After many weeks, my mom did start to show improvement, so she was allowed to return to the facility. She no longer stole food but had also lost weight. She also seemed confused and disinterested due to her new behavior medications.

As I celebrated Christmas in 2015, it was difficult to accept that my mom, who was present just last year at our home, would not be this year (and those to come). Our visit to San Luis Obispo, CA, for New Year's Eve brought memories of her with us at that location earlier in the year. I struggled as thoughts battled within. I experienced happiness with the freedom from being a direct caregiver but also sadness that my mom now resided in a memory-care facility. The guilt associated with the fact that I was the one who placed her there resurfaced, leaving me feeling as though I had abandoned her.

As I continued through that season, my stepdad passed away, and I became the primary decision-maker and advocate for my mother. As I was dealing with my grief over losing him, I was also battling with decisions regarding her care. I doubted my ability to make those choices. Every time her condition worsened, I wondered whether we would get through this next hurdle. I held my breath with every phone call as I waited to hear the latest issues and health concerns. Sometimes I still wonder why God puts up with my silliness and doubting. I often felt like Moses or the Israelites who, despite all of God's provisions and assurances, still questioned Him. I fluctuated between those cherished moments of strength and faith, and conflicting times of weakness and doubt. A huge lesson I learned was that I am not God. There are so many things about this life that I will probably never fully comprehend. I cannot handle it alone, nor am I called to do so. John 3:30 tells us that "He must become greater; I must become less." He just wants me to recognize that He is there; and that He will always be the constant, never-changing Lord of my life. Our God is bigger than any problem I can imagine or experience. He is indeed faithful.

By January 2016, my mother's decline was becoming more apparent. She needed a lot of prompting and physical assistance getting out of bed, toileting, and dressing. When asked if she wanted to go for a walk, she would just look at me with a blank stare. Whereas before she enjoyed sitting and watching television, now she would only do so if someone was sitting with her. She reverted once again to lying in bed for a significant portion of the day, so I had to push for staff to work at getting her up and attending activities. Different behaviors took the place of the previous ones but weren't as aggressive as before. These included flushing paper towels in the toilet due to her inability to understand that they belonged in the trash, thus flooding the restroom occasionally. She also exhibited stubbornness regarding taking walks.

Over the next few years, we saw numerous changes and an even more significant decline. Mom's body struggled with an auto-immune disorder on top of everything else. She constantly had sores that would not heal. Her dementia now caused behavior where she would bite and chew on her fingers, causing deep wounds. We tried many treatments, like wearing gloves and putting her in long-sleeve shirts, to no avail. In addition to these various ailments, she also had a bad fall and was sent to the hospital; as a result, she was very agitated, frightened, and confused, which necessitated the use of restraints. Due to what happened in the hospital, we were forced to make some difficult decisions regarding her subsequent care.

> *If you remain in me and my words remain in you, ask whatever you wish, and it will be done for you. This is to my Father's glory, that you bear much fruit, showing yourselves to be my disciples.* *John 15:7–8*

As I focused on this verse, I understood that as long as I am faithful to pray according to His will and read His word, He will answer because it is to His glory. As a result of my prayers and new knowledge, I will bear fruit, which will bring Him glory. It was a timely reminder that my caregiving efforts on my mother's behalf were evidence of trying to be obedient to Him. As difficult as the decisions were, I was honoring her and following Him. In addition, he provided strength and assurances through my husband and my uncle, who fully agreed with my decisions as we moved forward.

Should further hospitalization be required, we did not want her to be subjected to all the agitation and confusion again. Therefore, we asked that she just be made comfortable at the home when, or if, that time came. Unfortunately, a few years later, we had to agonizingly repeat the tough decisions we had previously made regarding her care. Mom had been experiencing continuous vomiting, so the staff at the facility mistakenly disregarded instructions that were in place and took her to the hospital again. While there, doctors explained that some of her body's systems were failing, and she would need various intravenous treatments and likely need to be intubated, etc. (something that we had already noted that she would not tolerate). She was not eating or responding to the interventions they had tried thus far, so we respectfully declined and started palliative care. We requested that she return to the comfort of her room at the facility. Despite being told she had a few days left, my mom rallied again and began eating and drinking with assistance. For almost another two years, she continued the battle against dementia.

I entitled this chapter "the long and winding road" because dementia is truly a long, long road with many twists and turns. Over eight years later, after Mom had begun to show signs of dementia, she was catatonic and barely acknowledged the presence of her first great-grandchild during one of our visits. As I sat with her, I longed for days a few years prior when she was feisty and combative. Watching her struggle and choke on her food to the point of now requiring only a liquid diet, I secretly hoped she would reach out, grab my food again, and be able to chew it as she had once so easily done. Then, as she showed no emotion, I hoped she would suddenly laugh and ask if it was time for "Vanna and the Wheel of Fortune!" This later entry from my journal illustrates the emotional battle that often accompanies those caring for loved ones with dementia.

*January 27, 2021*

*Tomorrow is Mom's birthday. I am so sad that she doesn't realize it. Even now, I wish for those moments, just a few years ago, when she at least clapped along and got excited as they sang "Happy Birthday" to her. Now, there are no smiles, clapping, or eating of cake. Sometimes, she doesn't even eat [anything]. Again, Lord, I ask why? Why is she going through this? Why do we have to watch her go through it? It's at these moments when I am vacillating between despair, anger, frustration, and sadness that I feel as though all I can do is trust that You hear me. You know her needs and are more capable than me of providing for them. I cannot know what she is feeling, hearing, seeing, or thinking, but You can. So, I continue to ask…wait…and trust.*

———————————————————*From my journal*

At this point in my caregiving journey with my mom, I readily understood its emotional effect on me. I wanted people to know the mom I had known most of my life. Besides immediate family and a few close friends, most people who saw her now only knew her as the frail, bedridden and unresponsive shell of a woman who no longer interacted with the world around her. These people didn't know what a capable, unstoppable force-to-be-reckoned-with she had once been. They weren't aware of the years she had devoted to not only caring for three members of her family with HD or the relentless effort she gave to advocating on their, and others, behalf. It was as if a huge chunk of her life never existed. Experiencing this saddened me and made dealing with dementia harder than just the daily care and advocacy required. I wrote this poem for Mother's Day as I sought to work through the myriad of emotions that consistently tugged at my heart.

*Mom,*

*Even though your mouth can no longer form the words I so long to hear,*
*I still cherish the memories of a mom who spoke the words I still hold dear.*

*Your eyes are fixed, and your look is now glazed,*
*But I fondly remember so many happier days*

*While I can no longer know what thoughts you may want to share with me,*
*I am, in part, the woman I am today because of all you shared and how you taught me to be.*

*Your arms no longer hold me in your tender loving embrace,*
*Yet I am proud that you are so strong and have run such a courageous race.*

*Your life was not an easy one, even before this season of life you are living now,*
*But you lived it with love, courage, strength, and hope that someday, somehow—*

*I would be able to lead a life free from all the sickness and disease that prevailed in our lives.*

*So thank you, Mom, for having that hope; for all the prayers prayed on my behalf; for all the sacrifices you made; and, most of all, for giving me life.*
*God answered your prayers, and you helped to create a legacy that is living on —as evidenced in the lives of your grandchildren and in the hearts and minds of a family that loves and appreciates you.*
*I love you now and always will.*

*Your daughter,*
*Lyndy*

After Mom's dementia had caused such deterioration that she was fully wheelchair-bound and often bedridden, she no longer required a locked unit. The staff at her facility asked that we consider relocating her to a different ward at the facility. It was yet another difficult decision for me to make because I felt like the change might be confusing to her. However, after being told of the immediate need for beds in the memory care unit where she was currently residing, we felt that it was best to allow them to relocate her. We decided to give another family the same opportunity we had received because we knew the agony of waiting for a spot in a facility that could address the many needs associated with dementia. Mom adjusted well to the new unit, and our family continued to visit as usual and take her on walks or little outings across the street for an ice cream treat.

January 2020 brought a pandemic, which vastly changed the way we were able to interact with my mom. For almost a year, we were only allowed to see her via FaceTime a few times a month. Eventually, we were allowed to visit in person, outdoors, where they would bring her out at an appointed time and seat her at least six feet from us. Unfortunately, these visits were relatively fruitless since she couldn't hear us from so far away and often couldn't even see us depending on how they positioned her chair. In addition, her body was significantly atrophied and rigid, so she had to be placed in the correct position for us even to see her face. As hard as it was to see her like this, I at least found joy in knowing she must have liked the sun's warmth on her face.

In July 2021, I received a call that mom was no longer eating and that she had lost a considerable amount of weight over a short period. We knew that her time on this earth was limited, so we jumped through all the Covid-related cautionary hoops to go and visit her for the brief amount of time allowed, not knowing that it would be the last. As I reflect on that day, I marvel at how God's hand was in the midst of it all. My husband and I were finally allowed to see her (after much confusion despite our visit being a preapproved "end-of-life" visit). She looked very peaceful as she was lying there in her bed. I quietly read some Bible verses aloud and told her how much we all loved her. I left that day feeling as though I was okay with that being the last time I would see her. I had prayed, over the years, that God would take her in her sleep, thus allowing me to escape having to be there in the end. It was tough to have been there when my sister and father died. Hence, I did not plan to return after that visit. Mom's brother arrived a few hours after my husband and I had left, and he stayed with her all afternoon and evening, holding her hand (something we had not been allowed to do because of time limits and social distancing, but for some reason he had been allowed to). I found out later that he had desired to be with her in the end, and he was. I received the call from him that evening that she had peacefully passed.

Now that the road had finally come to an "end," I had many conflicting emotions. Through all the years of being a caregiver as a young child/teen/adult and the later years of providing care and advocacy for my mother, I often felt that I just needed to get over the next hurdle and that one day it would all be over. It was like I was running a race with an eventual finish line. But then, I realized that, for so many years, I had been relying on my mom's strength. Later, I relied on my husband's strength. All the while, I was attempting to boost my inner sense of stability through others. With my mother's passing, I'm sure I thought I would feel an enormous weight lifted, but that was not the case. Instead, I had been slowly saying goodbye to my family members over the many years of dealing with the devastating diseases that ravaged their bodies, personalities, and minds. So, when the time came to say that final farewell, while bittersweet, it was not the overwhelming grief or relief I had anticipated. Instead, I had finally come to understand that it was my faith and the strength of God that ultimately enabled me to find joy amidst the pain and constant sorrow.

*Jesus, You alone are my defender and loving King*
*In Your love for me, You have given me everything.*

*You protect me even when I do not know*

*And are by my side wherever I go.*

*Thank You for your covenant offered and freely given to me*
*In which I am loved for all eternity.*

*Lyndy Downs*

# Conclusion

*For we are God's handiwork, created in Christ Jesus to do good works, which God prepared in advance for us to do.* *Ephesians 2:10*

I remember a puzzle of my Dad's that drove us crazy. It was a cherry pie, and every single piece looked identical. But, of course, each one was different and had a specific spot. As we progressed with placing each piece, we slowly began to see the image taking form. What was at first a jumbled mess now made complete sense. I am like one of those puzzle pieces in God's master puzzle, and I have learned that He knows how I fit and has a picture-perfect plan for each part of my life.

At the age of 58, I am the last living member of my original family of five, and with my mom's death, I feel an end of an era has come. However, I simultaneously sense the continuance of an awakening within me. Over the past 58 years, I have likely faced more challenges than the average person. I experienced love, joy, anger, sorrow, hardship, frustration, guilt, anxiety, and redemption. I have known what it felt like to be drowning in my endless sea of despair and doubt, yet saved by miraculous moments of strength and an assuredness that could only come from God.

Do I still struggle with those same emotions of yesteryear now that the "fight" against Huntington's Disease and dementia has ended in my family? Simply put, the answer is "yes." I find myself saddened and if I am honest, angry over all the "what ifs" associated with the loss created by the diseases that prevailed for so long in my life. There are those times when I wonder what my life would have been like had my sister and brother lived beyond their young adult years. What would it have been like to have siblings with whom I could share the good and bad times? Or who had the same faith? What kind of grandfather would my dad have been? What would it have been like to seek his help when I had financial issues? Could he have used his carpenter skills to help Rob with our remodeling? What would the joy on my mom's face look like as she met her great-grandchildren and we baked Christmas cookies together?

I still fear my sons won't remember their grandmother as the loving, capable woman she was for so much of their childhood, just as I could not remember my happier childhood years. Unfortunately, we are often robbed of sought-after joyful memories when dealing with long-term diseases. Fond recollections, that may have been generated over a duration of time longer than that of the presence of the disease, get lost amidst dealing with the everyday struggles and care warranted by the needs of the affected loved one.

I am concerned that instead of remembering the times Grandma accompanied us to various museums, parks, and other home-school field trips, that they will only recall the instances where they had to stop her from wandering off. Or perhaps they will forget about the special treats she would make for them and only be able to remember when they had to stop her from eating food or inedible items she wasn't supposed to eat. Maybe, instead of remembering how she lovingly cared for them when they would visit her house, they will only recall having to help her use the toilet when she could no longer do so herself.

But now, as I have learned to refocus those feelings,

my perspective has changed. I am convinced that it is during those moments of sorrow, worry, anxiety, and concern that I must choose to focus on the many blessings that I *know* have occurred. To dwell on the "*what if*" and "*what could have been*" thoughts precludes me from seeing the "*what God has done*" in my life occurrences. So, despite what memories my sons may have, I am confident that the Lord blessed the years spent with their grandma and created a lasting foundation. They may not recall specifics about Grandma's love and care for them, but because of that very same love she gave, they, in turn, showed love, concern, and compassion for her.

I have realized that all those years I so desperately wish I could regain in my memories, while not vivid, are still part of me. I have learned that my experience growing up with HD, though difficult, was the life God intended for me to live. It was a life in which He gave me the strength to thrive, and it is in living it that I have become who I am today. I am so grateful for the growth and change that has occurred inside me throughout these years, and I continue to seek to know more. Yet, one of the greatest lessons He has taught me in that quest is that I am not Him.

After all these years, comprehending that I am not God should be a reasonably basic concept. Yet, I have realized that I have spent much of my existence trying to be Him. I have lived as if my life was a giant Etch A Sketch drawing toy where I would draw lines attempting to achieve the picture-perfect result of how I felt things should be. Whenever I thought the drawing was nearing completion, something would shake it up, and I had to start all over again. I wanted so badly to be the one who would save my family from the awful effects of Huntington's Disease and dementia. If I just fought a little harder, I could escape the pain and suffering that I was enduring. So, I put on those "rose-colored" glasses in my attempt to see a "normal" life. But God, in His grace and mercy, was patient with me and helped me to see now that it was in my weakest moments that I was strong. During those heartfelt cries to Him, I experienced my greatest strength because He helped me understand that I needed to stop relying on myself and depend on Him.

*...so that your faith might not rest on human wisdom, but on God's power.* *1 Corinthians 2:5*

I now understand that it is that very dependence on Him that enabled me to make some of the most challenging decisions I have ever had to make. After much prayer and seeking God's wisdom, I learned to take "leaps of faith." In doing so, I surrendered to His sovereignty over my life and my family's. As a result, I became more able to realize how He was at work both in and through me. Finally, I could trust that He was in control despite my feelings that the walls were crumbling around me.

I'm continuously drawn to Him in my moments of despair. Instead of wringing my hands and focusing on all the things that could go wrong, I can see what He has done in my life thus far and be thankful. I have put away my rose-colored glasses and instead choose to use my magnifying glass so that I can see that—

> *...he said to me, 'My grace is sufficient for you, for my power is made perfect in weakness.' Therefore I will boast all the more gladly about my weaknesses, so that Christ's power may rest on me.* *2 Corinthians 12:9*

While I cannot know what lies ahead in the years I have left to live, I can now honestly praise Him for all

He has done and will continue to do in my life. I am confident that—

> *He must become greater; I must become less.*
>
> *John 3:30*

Only then do I see
His strength in me.

# NOTES

1. "Overview of Huntington's Disease." *Huntington's Disease Society of America*, 6 Nov. 2020, https://hdsa.org/what-is-hd/overview-of-huntingtons-disease/.

2. "Juvenile Onset HD" *Huntington's Disease Society of America*, 23 May 2019, https://hdsa.org/what-is-hd/history-and-genetics-of-huntingtons-disease/juvenile-onset-hd/.

3. "The Genetics of Juvenile Huntington's Disease" *Huntington's Disease Association*, 23 Mar. 2018, https://www.hda.org.uk/huntingtons-disease/what-is-juvenile-huntingtons-disease/genetics-of-juvenile-huntingtons-disease.

4. Gusella, James F. "A Polymorphic DNA Marker Genetically Linked to Huntington's Disease." *Nature*, vol. 306, no. 17, Nov. 1983, p. 234.

5. Giglio, Louie. *Goliath Must Fall: Winning the Battle Against Your Giants*, Thomas Nelson, 2017, pg. 74

6. "Frontotemporal Dementia." *Mayo Clinic, Mayo Foundation for Medical Education and Research*, 16 Nov. 2021, https://www.mayoclinic.org/diseases-conditions/frontotemporal-dementia/symptoms-causes/syc-20354737.

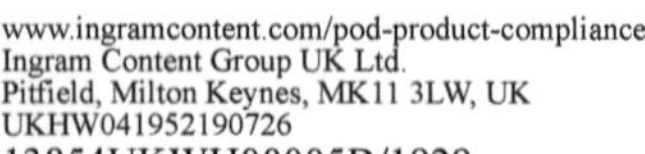
www.ingramcontent.com/pod-product-compliance
Ingram Content Group UK Ltd.
Pitfield, Milton Keynes, MK11 3LW, UK
UKHW041952190726
13854UKWH00005B/1929

9 798218 093211